Midwifery, Mind and Spirit

Midwifery, Mind and Spirit:
Emerging issues of care

Jennifer Hall MSc RN RM ADM

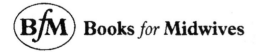 **Books** *for* **Midwives**

OXFORD   AUCKLAND   BOSTON   JOHANNESBURG   MELBOURNE   NEW DELHI

Books for Midwives
An imprint of Butterworth-Heinemann
Linacre House, Jordan Hill, Oxford OX2 8DP
225 Wildwood Avenue, Woburn, MA 01801–2041
A division of Reed Educational and Professional Publishing Ltd

℞ A member of the Reed Elsevier plc group

First published 2001

© Jennifer Hall 2001

British Library Cataloguing in Publication Data
A catalogue record for this book is available from the British Library

Library of Congress Cataloguing in Publication Data
A catalogue record for this book is available from the Library of
Congress

ISBN 0 7506 4297 1

Composition by Genesis Typesetting, Rochester, Kent
Printed and bound in Great Britain

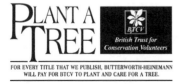

FOR EVERY TITLE THAT WE PUBLISH, BUTTERWORTH-HEINEMANN
WILL PAY FOR BTCV TO PLANT AND CARE FOR A TREE.

RG
526
H35
2001

Contents

This book is dedicated to my daughters, Katie, Beth, Maddie, Abigail and Isobel, who all arrived at various times during the development of this book, and so have fed into the ideas and thought processes just by being there.

My hope is that, by the time they get to the age of giving birth, it will be a spiritual event and not the product of a technological revolution.

To the memory of Marlies Brooks (1960–2000) who informed the original study for this book, but will never have the chance to read it.

Introduction

Spiritual issues have been the taboo subjects of the 1990s. If we had lived in the Victorian era the taboo would have been sex; around the war years until the 1970s it may have been death. But now it appears we have problems discussing anything related to things that are not tangible, that cannot be demonstrated through research. Talking to colleagues about the subject of this book produced a variety of reactions. The cynical sly smile was one, indicating a belief in my insanity at even daring to mention it! There were others who were embarrassed and more that were obviously pretending to be interested. Others too have been as passionate about the topic as me and provided valuable information through their insights.

But why write a book on such a controversial subject? Primarily, because I believe that someone has to start the debate for midwives. In nursing in recent years there have been moves towards giving holistic care. Holism in the general sense has been given the meaning 'whole' or 'complete', with the understanding that a person is a combination of body, mind and spirit (e.g. Stoll, 1979; Labun, 1988; Price *et al.*, 1995). However, there is an argument that separating a person into these three parts is contradictory to the aims of an holistic or complete approach (Goddard, 1995). Though generally the physical and emotional aspects of care are acknowledged, it is argued that the spiritual aspects may still be neglected (Ross, 1994; Price *et al.*, 1995; McSherry, 1996). A contrast may be noted between the historical practices of midwives and nurses and the influence of spirituality, and the position today, where science and technology have the greater influence (Cusveller, 1998). Recently the nursing press has given space to nurses' discussions of the spiritual aspects of care (see, for example, various articles in the *Nursing Times* from July 1997 to January 1998) and, among the public, a greater awareness of spiritual matters developed as the new millennium approached. In these issues, nurses are further on than midwives.

From a personal view, this book has evolved from my experience as a midwife, where I was aware that the experiences of individual women appeared to be enhanced by the presence of particular midwives. This caused me to ask what it was about these midwives that enabled them to give such special care to the women. The recognition that many of these midwives also had some form of spiritual belief led me to question whether the two were connected.

My own experience of pregnancy and childbirth and the changes I have experienced in myself have led me to continue the questioning process. The relationship with each child has been unique and special from the moment of conception, and continues now as I am their mother. I am aware that my spiritual journey began long before the arrival of the children, and I question how much such a journey has an effect on the birthing experience of the individual. I know, too, that my experience was enhanced by the loving care of a truly spiritual midwife. For the last two births, though apart by many miles, the care was given over the telephone and through the postal system! I acknowledge, too, that my spiritual journey has been encouraged and grown through the love and support of my husband, who recognizes my worth and significance as a woman first, and mother second.

For midwives in the UK, holistic care is written into the rules of practice, with the assumption that midwifery education will give: '... the ability to assess, plan, implement and evaluate care within the sphere of practice of a midwife to meet the physical, emotional, social, spiritual and educational needs of the mother and baby and the family.' (UKCC, 1993, p. 13).

I believe it is debatable that midwifery education is enabling students and practitioners meet the spiritual needs of the mother and her family. There has been no article relating to the subject in British professional midwifery journals within the past 20 years, and spirituality and spiritual care are omitted from the mainstream midwifery textbooks. In contrast, such issues have been explored by women in their capacities as mothers, lay carers and feminists, indicating that the subject is of relevance to women (Hebblethwaite, 1984; Stockley, 1986; Achterberg, 1990; King, 1993). As there is a lack of academic work relating to spiritual issues associated with midwifery practice, it has been appropriate to approach this book using the work of nurses, other health workers and women, worldwide.

In the light of the knowledge that midwives so far have failed to address the issues of spirituality in the context of birth and midwifery practice, this book intends to be a beginning. One aim is that it will open the door to discussion and lead on to the issues being taken seriously and researched in order to gain credibility in academic disciplines. Throughout each chapter there are a number of questions which may be used for the purpose of personal study or as a source for discussion. Another aim is that the book will provide a source from which educationalists can teach others and from which those from religious disciplines can gain understanding of some of the birth processes in order to provide a woman with support during her pregnancy. I do not suggest that it will provide all the answers, but I am hoping that it will leave the reader with some questions and a desire to debate the issues further with others.

Reflective questions

1 How do I react when 'spirituality' is mentioned?
2 Do I give spiritual care now?
3 How do I feel about discussing spiritual matters?

Acknowledgements

I am indebted and grateful to a number of people for their support in preparing this book:

To Sandy Kirkman – as supervisor of the original review, she has become a mentor and friend, and has informed this book with truly spiritual wisdom by reading initial draft chapters.

To Philip Burnard – who kindly took time out of a busy schedule to encourage me to write this in the first place and read draft chapters.

To the librarians of UWCM and Ann Brown at Trinity College, Bristol – for her help and encouragement.

To my friends and family at Henleaze and Westbury Community Church, Bristol – for all the support and love given, which ranged from prayer to child care. Thank you.

To Jenny Fraser – a truly spiritual midwife and a dear friend, who always gets me thinking.

To our parents – for continued love and practical help.

To Susan Devlin and Mary Seager at Butterworth-Heinemann – for being willing to go with the idea and provide excellent editorial support.

To Katie, Beth and Maddie – for being so patient with a preoccupied mum.

And finally, my most heartfelt thanks go to my husband, Mark – without him this would not have been written. He has been my support financially, physically and spiritually, giving up much of our 'normal' life, including a lot of his time, in and out of work, to provide child care. He has always made me feel loved and valued and has believed alongside me that this project has been worth the sacrifices. Truly he has been my 'Mr Motivator'. Thanks.

1 *Spirituality and spiritual care*

According to the rules of practice outlined in the introduction, it is expected that spiritual care will be an integral part of the holistic care given by midwives. But what does spirituality and spiritual care mean and how may they be incorporated as a dimension of midwifery practice?

Reflection: Before continuing answer the question 'what do spirituality and spiritual care mean to you?'.

Definitions of spirituality

Unfortunately the defining of such issues is a complex matter, due to the multifactorial elements involved (see Table 1.1). The process of isolating these elements leads to the question of whether the presence of just one is evidence of spirituality or whether there has to be a combination of them all. Also, can spirituality be explored in isolation from the rest of a person's physical and emotional self? Studying the available literature reveals that there is a lack of consistency in presenting a definition of the concepts. One writer simplifies it to being a 'journey towards inner peace' (Brown, 1998) while another has suggested that personal wholeness is necessary to demonstrate spiritual integrity (Labun, 1988). This wholeness is also likely to be expressed in an individual way, and is suggested to be affected by cultural background, how a person is brought up and by the social structure in which they live (Cawley, 1997). The interrelational aspects of the mind, body and spirit are also acknowledged, as is the fact that the spiritual dimension appears to have a relationship with health and well-being (e.g. Moberg, 1979; Waugh, 1992; Daaleman *et al.*, 1994; Price *et al.*, 1995).

If these concepts are placed in the context of midwifery, the indication is that we should acknowledge the relationship of the mind, body and spirit to the changes taking place within the woman during the time surrounding pregnancy and birth. Also we should explore how the spiritual dimension has a relationship with the health and well-being of the woman and child.

Table 1.1   Elements of spirituality

---

1. *Transcendence*: concept of something beyond this worldly existence, i.e. supernatural, or aspiring to know more in terms of personal meaning.

Lane (1987)	Kaye and Robinson (1994)
Labun (1988)	Praill (1995)
Stoll (1989)	Price *et al.* (1995)
Waugh (1992)	Amenta (1997)
	O'Shea (1998)

2. *Search for meaning and purpose*

Fish and Shelley (1978)	King (1993)
Highfield and Cason (1983)	Sims (1994)
Burnard (1988)	Burkhardt (1994)
Labun (1988)	Praill (1995)
Simsen (1988)	Price *et al.* (1995)
Waugh (1992)	Amenta (1997)
	O'Shea (1998)

3. *Belonging/connecting*: desiring to belong to something, someone, somewhere.

Lane (1987)	Sims (1994)
Burkhardt (1994)	Tucakovic (1994)
	O'Shea (1998)

4. *Relational aspects*: doing for others, giving life and love, receptive of love, having trust and forgiveness.

Dickinson (1975)	Stoll (1989)
Fish and Shelley (1978)	Waugh (1992)
Highfield and Cason (1983)	Burkhardt (1994)
Lane (1987)	Praill (1995)
Labun (1988)	Amenta (1997)
	O'Shea (1998)

5. *Self-awareness*: self-worth, freedom to have and seek choices, creativity.

Lane (1987)	Price *et al.* (1995)
Stoll (1989)	McSherry (1996)
Burkhardt (1994)	Amenta (1997)
Tucakovic (1994)	O'Shea (1998)

6. *Hope and faith*

Fish and Shelley (1978)	Waugh (1992)
Highfield and Cason (1983)	Harrison and Burnard (1993)
Labun (1988)	Amenta (1997)
Stoll (1989)	O'Shea (1998)

Religious belief

It would appear that to many people the concept of spirituality is involved with a particular religion. Within health care this confines history-taking to discovering the affiliation of the client, usually to a particular denomination rather than religious persuasion, without assessing the level of the person's belief (Stoll, 1979; Sims, 1994). It is suggested that a religious view is very limiting and may lead to:

- Conflict between the differences in faith of the patient and carer.
- Guilt within the person related to their religious belief.
- Leaving it to the religious 'experts' rather than recognizing spirituality in every person (Edassery and Kuttierath, 1998).

It is appropriate to recognize the value placed on organized religious practices and rituals to some, and the meanings gained from them (Stoll, 1979; McGilloway, 1985; Allen, 1991; Schott and Henley, 1996). However, the definitions of spirituality indicate a wider concept of belief and meaning than just religion, that embraces those who have no religious belief (McGilloway, 1985; Burnard, 1988; Harrison *et al.,* 1993; Price *et al.,* 1995; Cawley, 1997). It has been suggested that every person looks for something or someone on which to focus worship, and this could be a personal God, another person or an object (Stoll, 1989). Waugh (1992) suggests there are vertical and horizontal dimensions to spirituality. She indicates that the vertical dimension is the relationship with God, either in or out of religion, or it 'may constitute the individual's value system which forms the focus of their life' (p. 8). The vertical dimension is thus an individual's personal motivations for life's meaning and significance (Stoll, 1989). Waugh (1992) presents the horizontal dimension as how the person reflects and reacts to the transcendent relationship or level of self-actualization through their way of living and their relationships with themselves, other people and their environment. These two dimensions thus constitute a person's spirituality: how they express spirituality on a personal level and how this is then transferred to living within the world around.

Within that framework, Waugh (1992, p. 10) suggests a definition of spirituality as '... that element within man, from which originates: meaning, purpose and fulfillment in life; a will to live; belief and faith in self, others and God, and which is essential to the attainment of an optimum state of well-being, health or quality of life'.

This definition provides a broad structure from which the elements of spirituality may be discussed as appropriate to pregnancy and birth. However, it should be noted that the definition fails to acknowledge the suggestion that women's experiences of expressing spirituality are different to those of men (King, 1989; Burkhardt, 1994). It will be appropriate to discuss such issues due to the uniquely feminine aspects of childbirth.

Reflection: Does the definition of spirituality above reflect closely your own beliefs?

Spiritual care

To provide spiritual care is to be able to assess the spiritual needs of the client and to be able to meet those needs. Waugh (1992, p. 248) suggests that spiritual nursing care should be to aim at '. . . putting the patient in the best condition for the spiritual realm to act upon him'.

Reflection: Is this what spiritual care means to you? Can you identify what the writer means by the above statement?

Table 1.2 provides a list of the elements of spiritual care identified from other writers.

It has been suggested that it is essential for a nurse to have self-awareness, with or without religious belief, or she will be unable to give effective spiritual care (Carson, 1989a). Others have highlighted that there is a need for carers to be aware of their own beliefs, and why they have them, in order to be able to recognize the spiritual needs in others (Corrine *et al.*, 1992; Harrison and Burnard, 1993). It is also suggested that a carer's belief will be influential on how she makes decisions and prioritizes care (Cusvellar, 1998). From this it could be viewed that recognition of personal belief is essential for a spiritual carer.

Waugh's study (1992) investigating nurses' perceptions of how they perceived spiritual need and care, and how they gave it, showed that the nurses' personal characteristics are relevant. She ascertained that those who had an awareness of spiritual care:

- Had an awareness of their own spirituality.
- Were searching for meaning in their own lives.
- Had experienced some form of personal crisis.
- Recognized spiritual care as part of their role.
- Had sensitive and perceptive traits.
- 'Were able to identify a broader range of spiritual needs and give spiritual care at a deeper level than those who did not demonstrate these characteristics' (pp. 236–237).

There are indications that there may be some form of beneficial spiritual growth taking place within those who give care (Kaye and Robinson, 1994; Brown, 1998). Gaskin (1977) goes further by indicating that a midwife should have a spiritual belief, as each birth is regarded as a 'holy' event. She suggests the midwife will be unable to provide complete care without living a spiritual life. Those midwives without beliefs may take offence at

Table 1.2   Elements of spiritual care

---

1. *Recognizing value and acceptance of each person*

    Dickinson (1975)   Allen (1991)
    Gaskin (1977)   Burkhardt (1994)
    Labun (1988)   Price *et al.* (1995)

2. *Giving support/having presence*: 'being there'.

    Dickinson (1975)   Praill (1995)
    Harrison and Burnard (1993)   Price *et al.* (1995)
                                               McSherry (1996)

3. *Self-awareness*

    Dickinson (1975)   Allen (1991)
    Myco (1985)   Waugh (1992)
    Labun (1988)   Price *et al.* (1995)
                                               McSherry (1996)

4. *Understanding*

    Dickinson (1975)   Burkhardt (1994)
    Labun (1988)   Price *et al.* (1995)
                                               McSherry (1996)

5. *Openness/using intuition*

    Dickinson (1975)   Waugh (1992)
    Gaskin (1977)   Harrison and Burnard (1993)
    Allen (1991)   Price *et al.* (1995)
                                               Davis-Floyd and Davis (1997)

6. *Willingness to help others find meaning*

    Dickinson (1975)   Harrison and Burnard (1993)
    Fish and Shelley (1978)   Burkhardt (1994)
    Labun (1988)   Praill (1995)
    Simsen (1988)   Price *et al.* (1995)
    Waugh (1992)   McSherry (1996)

7. *Counselling skills*
    Fish and Shelley (1978)   Burkhardt (1994)
    Labun (1988)   Praill (1995)
    Harrison and Burnard (1993)   McSherry (1996)

8. *Love and compassion*
    Gaskin (1977)   Waugh (1992)
    Fish and Shelley (1978)

---

such a statement and yet prior to the Middle Ages, it is known that midwives played a spiritual role in labour care (McCool and McCool, 1989; Achterberg, 1990). It is suggested that midwives became silent about their role in spiritual matters 'in order for midwifery to survive as a profession' (Achterberg, 1990). Achterberg further suggests that, although being a midwife was not seen as being an 'honourable position', it was a powerful one, because the established Church tried to keep control of the practices.

Reflection: What is your response to the suggestion that midwives should have some form of spiritual belief in order to give spiritual care?

Recent research into how women perceive the caring role of the midwife indicates that women recognize the importance of the presence of many of the elements of spiritual care (see Table 1.3 and Berg *et al.*, 1996). Some midwives also use prayer, incantations or rituals as interventions in labour care (Wagner, 1995; Penwell, 1996; Kitzinger, 1997), which indicates that some have a recognition of spiritual elements within birth. Cusveller (1995) argues that nurses with religious commitment have a particular bias in the care they give. Though there is no evidence to suggest the same may be applicable to midwives, both psychiatrists and nurses have stated the need to have awareness of personal beliefs and to acknowledge how they may affect practice, but not to impose those beliefs on those within their

Table 1.3 Traits of the caring nurse-midwife

Trait	Demonstrated by: _____
Competence	Knowledge and skills Responsible attitude Attentiveness Deliberate and determined actions Effective communication
Genuine concern and respect for the woman	Giving of her- or himself Solidarity and sharing Encouragement and support Respect Benevolence
Positive mental attitude	Cheerfulness Positive attitude Reliability Trustworthiness Being considerate and understanding.

Source: Halldorsdottir *et al.* (1996).

care (Burnard, 1988; Allen, 1991; Sims, 1994). However, there is a lack of provision of educational programmes for midwives that include spiritual matters as part of the curriculum, though it is a need recognized by nursing educationalists (Waugh, 1992; Harrison and Burnard, 1993; Narayana-samy, 1993; Ross, 1996).

Spiritual distress

Education surrounding spiritual care should also include the ability to recognize spiritual distress. In America this is classified as a Nursing Diagnosis (Stoll, 1979), and has been suggested to be: '. . . the state in which the individual experiences, or is at risk of experiencing, a disturbance in the belief or value system that provides strength, hope and meaning to life' (Carpenito, 1993 cited by Price *et al.*, 1995). Waugh (1992, p. 14) defines spiritual distress as: 'the state resulting when an individual is deprived of having their spiritual needs fulfilled'.

A sign of distress may be a demonstrated anger towards God or a conflict in respect of the person's faith (Sumner, 1998). However, other elements include questioning a meaning for existence, a sense of meaninglessness or hopelessness, a feeling of alienation or aloneness, and changes of behaviour, such as crying, withdrawal and anger (Burnard, 1988; Waugh, 1992; Harrison and Burnard, 1993). A more recent phenomenological study investigating spiritual distress in ten subjects who had experienced anxieties 'about the meaning of life, death, and/or beliefs' (Smucker, 1996), described two distinct phases in the development of the condition. The first phase related to a particular event that 'suddenly or unexpectedly breaks into one's life' and the second was described as 'rebuilding' (Smucker 1996). Within the first phase the researcher isolated the themes of falling apart, wondering or questioning, and recognizing 'something beyond'. In the second phase were the themes of stability, change and growth, wondering in awe at the mystery of life, and the 'something beyond' becoming more of a central part of the person's life. The researcher concludes that: '. . . the presence of a second phase, which evolved out of spiritual distress for these participants, may indicate that spiritual distress is more than a problem. It also may hold the potential for spiritual growth' (p. 89).

Spiritual distress may therefore develop in situations where questions of belief and meaning follow stressful life events (Harrison and Burnard, 1993), but it may also have a more positive result for some, if the above research could be applied to a wider population. This is applicable to midwifery, where stressful situations take place and distress may develop, not only in the client but also in the partner (Corrine *et al.*, 1992; Brown, 1993; Smucker, 1996).

Distress may also occur in the caring midwife (Harrison and Burnard, 1993). Intensive caring and giving out may lead to spiritual distress, as well as being physically and emotionally draining, and it is appropriate for the midwife to recognize this in herself, as well as in others. It is significant that Waugh (1992) completed her study by advocating adequate staffing levels for spiritual care to take place effectively. Adequate levels should also ensure protection of the carer's spiritual self from 'burn-out' (Fish and Shelley, 1978).

Spiritual midwifery care

Spiritual care, as discussed in this chapter, is being able to assess the spiritual needs of a client and then meeting those needs. It could be argued that this is unlikely to be taking place via midwives at the present time, as there is so little spiritual awareness documented in midwifery texts. Where midwifery care is cited in spiritual terms words are used such as trust, faith, support, respect, honour, empowerment, flexibility, love, talking, touch, prayer, positive thinking, compassion, openness, instinct, individualized care, sensitivity and encouragement (Gaskin, 1977; Edmunds, 1995; Rawlings, 1995; Wagner, 1995; Page, 1996; Kitzinger, 1997).

The majority of these words are used to describe midwifery care generally. This indicates that it is possible that midwives are already undertaking spiritual care without naming it as such. In this respect, the elements of spiritual care described in Table 1.2 will be explored in relation to the care given by midwives. The need for suitable assessment is necessary for the provision of appropriate spiritual care, and therefore the process of assessment by midwives will also be explored in relation to giving this care.

> *Reflection: In your opinion, are all midwives already giving spiritual care, are some of them or none at all? Do you believe you give spiritual care and what does this mean to you?*

Assessment

As in any form of care, it would appear that appropriate assessment needs to be carried out if spiritual care is to be effective. Many carers believe spirituality is limited to involvement with a particular religion, which means that history-taking is confined to discovering the affiliation of the client without assessing the level and meaning of the person's belief (Stoll, 1979; Corrine *et al.*, 1992; Waugh, 1992; Narayanasamy, 1993; Sims, 1994; Oldnall, 1996; Brown-Saltzman, 1997).

> *Reflection: Do you believe spirituality is confined to those having religious belief or involvement?*

Assessment tools

Within nursing practice tools for assessing spiritual need and the audit of spiritual care are already being developed. In North America, for example, an assessment tool to identify spiritual distress is used (NANDA, 1994). More recently, the work carried out and demonstrated by the Trent Hospice Audit Group (Catterall *et al.*, 1998) showed how a simple questionnaire and verbal rating scale could be used to evaluate patients' feelings about their spiritual needs. From this they developed a standard for spiritual care within the hospice setting to enable further evaluation to take place. Within midwifery as yet we have no such tools, and research will need to be carried out to assess whether the ones used in nursing could be effectively carried across for use in midwifery practice.

The booking interview

During pregnancy the first time a woman encounters a midwife is usually at a booking interview. Within the format of most maternity notes is a question regarding the religion of the woman. Though to some people their religion is important, to others who have no belief this question could be embarrassing (Burnard, 1988), which may lead them to reply that they belong to the 'Church of England', which is a denomination of Christianity, and not a specific religion. Those with a strong faith may name the religion, as opposed to a denominational branch. It is argued that carers are not asking the right questions and that there should be a form of assessment to identify specific spiritual needs (Harrison and Burnard, 1993; Sims, 1994). However, the lack of formal research into the spirituality of pregnancy and birth means we are unsure which questions should be asked. Stoll (1979) and Carson (1989a) both advocate that any history should include:

- The person's concept of God or deity.
- The person's source of strength and hope.
- The significance of religious practices and ritual.
- The person's perceived relationship between his or her spiritual beliefs and state of health.

Burkhardt's (1994) study of women's spirituality suggested that assessment should include information on:

- How the woman perceives she fits into her world.
- The meanings she attaches to her life's events.
- Areas where she has experienced peace or had difficulties.
- How she is in touch with her inner self.
- What she does or where she goes to feel 'nurtured' and in touch with her self.

She also recommends enabling a woman to tell her story and that the carer should be focussed on being with and getting to know the woman. Such issues may be too daunting to explore within the confines and time limitations of a booking interview.

Reflection: How may a booking interview be expanded to include these issues? Do you feel the booking interview is the place for such a discussion?

Relationship

Labun (1988) suggests that the sensitivity of the subject requires the discussion to take place within a trusting relationship, and McSherry (1996) regards it as a continual process. This would imply that such issues may be better explored by a known midwife, once a relationship has developed. Within our culture it is indicated that spiritual issues may be too emotionally charged to allow immediate exploration (Stoll, 1979), and yet the embarrassment may come more from the carer than from the client (Simsen, 1986). Difficulties in understanding and communication may also make it hard to establish the client's spiritual needs (Ross, 1997). It has also been demonstrated that nurses are less likely to attempt spiritual assessment in situations where patents are acutely ill (Boutell and Bozett, 1990).

Reflection: Would you feel embarrassed about asking questions to do with spirituality? Why?

Continuity of care by midwives may place them in a better position to recognize the place of spirituality and religion in women's lives. Religious books, artefacts or mementos may be significantly placed in the home, and could be used as trigger points for conversation. Cultural differences should also be recognized in order to provide the best support for all aspects of care (Corrine *et al.*, 1992; Callister *et al.*, 1996; Morgan, 1996; Schott and Henley, 1996; Khalaf and Callister, 1997). It would also be appropriate to be aware of the resources and spiritual supports that are available in the local community, in order to recommend referral should it be required (Corrine *et al.*, 1992).

Reflection: Do you know what spiritual resources are available in your client's community?

The midwife should recognize that certain issues can hold spiritual significance for pregnant women. For instance:

- Infertility treatment (Duncan, 1993 cited by Guinness, 1993; Guinness, 1993; Harris, 1994).

- Fetal abnormality (Philps, 1991 cited by Guinness, 1993; Diachuk, 1994).
- Miscarriage (Stockley, 1986).
- Previous termination of pregnancy (Hall, 1990; Marck, 1994).

Any midwifery assessment should therefore include appropriate and sensitive questioning regarding these issues. As already discussed, the changes of pregnancy may cause the woman to evaluate previous beliefs. This may not be immediate, but at any time within the pregnancy, which would indicate that there is a need for continual assessment in order to be able to meet those needs.

Reflection: Have you been aware of particular situations or life experiences that have been particularly spiritually significant for women?

Conclusion

From the above information it is not possible to establish a definitive meaning for spirituality and spiritual care in midwifery. It is apparent, however, that there are elements that have been identified which have relevance, and in the following chapters these will be discussed within the context of midwifery care.

2 *Feminine spirituality*

Bearing and nurturing children is regarded as primarily a female role. The majority of midwives are also women. The fact that these statements have been written indicates some assumptions:

- That being female is different to being male.
- That being female is important to childbearing.

The first assumption may be debated, as, despite physical differences, persons from both genders may display a mixture of masculine and feminine characteristics. The second assumption is also debated by fathers, male carers and sociologists. Despite these debates, within this context it seems appropriate to discuss the feminine side of spirituality without negating men's expression of spiritual issues or their experiences of childbirth. It is important to emphasize that this chapter intends to focus on feminine, rather than feminist, spirituality, as the latter conjures up a more political framework instead of one which may be applicable to all women (King, 1993). However, much has been written about spiritual issues in recent years by women who profess to feminist views and therefore it will be appropriate to include reference to some of these.

It is of value to note that it has been suggested that the use of the word feminine is an emphasis on women's 'otherness' to men, so that women then view themselves as 'objects' rather than 'subjects' (King, 1993). It could be argued, however, that femininity is not a negative trait, and that both women and men should begin to see its worth in the context of our complex make-up. Therefore the aim is to use the word positively within this exploration.

> *Reflection: Reflect on what your thoughts were when you read the statements at the beginning of this chapter about childbearing. What are your understandings of the words female, feminine and feminist?*

Gender and spirituality

What is feminine spirituality? In reality, this is an unanswered question. It is notable that the majority of present health care research relating to spiritual issues does not distinguish between the genders of the study population, making the evaluation of such studies problematic. This would imply that the elements identified from research in Table 1.1 may be assumed to be relevant to the experiences of both women and men. Some feminist writers may argue that this would not be the case, as such research may have been carried out in a patriarchal way and has thus viewed women's experiences from a man's perspective. It is suggested that women's spirituality should be '... studied from the perspective of women's experience and within the context of their situation in time, in history and in culture' (Dobbie, 1991, p. 825).

Others have argued against an approach that seeks to identify specific female elements to spiritual belief. Hunt (1995) suggests there should be a process of 'feministization' in religion to prevent gender stereotyping. This may be valid, in that women will exhibit both masculine and feminine characteristics (as do men). From this it would appear appropriate to develop an individual approach to each person in order to meet their spiritual needs.

Feminine characteristics

Feminine characteristics from ancient societies have been identified, such as those of:

- Caring
- Compassion
- Non-violence
- Power to 'create and nurture life'
- Unity with 'Mother Earth'
- Wholeness
- Intuition (Tucakovic, 1994).

Intuitive 'knowing' is also suggested to be a particularly feminine trait by some authors (Estes, 1992; Harrison, 1993; Burkhardt, 1994; Davis, 1995; Davis-Floyd and Davis, 1997), while others have condemned intuition as being a trait with which women have been labelled to imply a lack in their reasoning abilities (Annandale and Clark, 1996).

King (1993) also highlights particular spiritual attributes within women. She states these to be:

- Suffering as a source of strength
- Attention to detail
- Faithfulness
- Listening

- Selfless giving
- Caring concern
- Adaptability to people
- Encouraging love
- Peacemakers
- Being earth or creation centred.

King also argues that women are more likely to view spirituality as being something that is intertwined with all aspects of life. In this respect, Rhodes (1997) views women's spirituality as being something that is 'integrated into a communal experience', something that is shared with others but is also part of the woman's 'primal feminine energy'.

Reflection: What are your responses to these suggestions of feminine attributes and characteristics?

Some researchers have attempted to establish elements that are unique to women's experiences (Burkhardt, 1994). In this study, the fact that only women were interviewed in a specific small area of Southern America, and not the men, indicates that any particular cultural variables have not been excluded nor has it been proven that these elements are specifically those of the feminine. With that criticism in mind, the fact that the women have shared their own experiences gives credence to the idea that what they discuss are 'women's' experiences – though they may not be exclusively those of women or of women of every culture. The study illustrated the way women express spirituality through telling their stories – an issue which has also been identified by other writers (Estes, 1992; King, 1993; O'Shea, 1998). The study also identified belonging and connecting relationships as being particularly important to this group of women.

Though this was a study of women's experiences, it is not known how exclusive these experiences are to women. Certainly searching for meaning is an integral part of most investigations into spiritual belief for both genders, and there is no doubt that men experience connecting relationships with God and other people. It is not known how much the intensity of these connecting relationships may be different in men and women or whether the story-telling aspect is as important for men.

Feminist spirituality

Ursula King's (1993) critique of feminism and spiritual issues provides an insight into some of the variety of understandings and experiences of women with feminist views. Her extensive review explores feminist thought through:

- Protest and anger at women's subordination in society.
- Challenging institutions, such as religion, role and status and language.
- Women's experiences of religion, global experiences, society and work, body existence and self.
- Women's experiences of spiritual power in history and mysticism.
- Investigation of new experiences of spirituality, including goddess worship and witchcraft, and concepts of androgyny.
- Investigation into new understandings of theology, including Christian belief through feminist views.
- Dimensions relating to ecology, peace and a worldwide perspective.

This highlights the diversity of approach through which feminists seek to explore or experience spirituality and consequently demonstrates that this diversity will be the same for all women. Sered (1994) also identifies the acceptance of individual women's experiences as legitimate as being at the core of 'spiritual feminism' as well as the political and witchcraft connections mentioned above. To define a particular feminine way of experiencing spirituality is therefore difficult, and reinforces the requirement to address spiritual need on an individual basis.

Reflection: What are your views on the dimensions of feminist spirituality as indicated above? Can men have these spiritual thoughts as well?

The elements of spirituality identified from various studies and presented in Table 1.1 provide a framework from which some of the issues for women may be determined.

Transcendence

A dictionary definition suggests the meaning of transcendent as: 'excelling, surpassing; transcending human experience' or '(esp. of God) existing apart from, not subject to limitations of, the material universe' (Sykes, 1977). Some writers have assumed that a transcendental relationship with God is an essential component of spiritual awareness (Stoll, 1977; Fish and Shelley, 1978; Stoll, 1989). However, transcending has also been defined as: 'the desire to step beyond who and what people are, aspiring to be something and know something more, to love more and create more' (Harrison *et al.*, 1993, p. 8 after Lane, 1987).

Thus, for the non-believer, transcendence may be related to a greater desire for an awareness beyond the limitations of physical boundaries.

Reflection: Are you able to identify your own beliefs?

Religious transcendence

Women have been shown to demonstrate more religious behaviour than men, especially in situations of serious life events (Reed, 1986). There are a number of religions where women play a greater role than men but there are no religions which can be described as 'typical' for women or men (Sered, 1994). The reasons for a person's particular choices about types of religious involvement appear to be manifold. Historically, the development of religion and religious practices has generally taken place in the context of men's beliefs in the western world. However, it is worth noting the existence of religions, primarily in Eastern areas of the world, where historically women have been the main participants and remain so today (Sered, 1994). Sered states that primary women's religions tend to be in societies where:

- Women control important resources.
- Families focus on mothers.
- Kinship ties are through the maternal line.

Ritual celebration of motherhood is common in societies where the mother role is viewed as more important over the role of wife. However, Sered (1994) states that in male-dominated religions women tend to be related to as wives or daughters.

It is only recently that women have been included within the leadership of the mainstream churches within the western world and subsequently allowed to study theology academically (King, 1993; Rhodes, 1997). Some women have purposefully removed themselves from such structured religion where patriarchal dominance is seen to be present, either because of the masculine portrayal of God as 'Father' or 'King', or because males are dominant, authoritarian figures within that religion (Storkey, 1985; Rich, 1992; King, 1993; Sered, 1994). Ironically, within these groups there tend to be more women worshippers (King, 1993; Hunt, 1995), though they are likely to hold positions of authority in less institutional religions (King, 1993).

As an alternative, rather than rejecting the traditional religions, some are developing within it a female theology (Hebblethwaite, 1984; Soskice, 1992; King, 1993; Sered, 1994; Rhodes, 1997). This is not just reflected within the Judaeo-Christian expressions but also in the other mainstream religions. Complications arise with respect to women's desires to express their femininity in religions where cultural expectations are also entwined. Different values may be placed on men and women within these cultures, undermining women's sense of self worth (Singh Kalsi, 1994; Yao, 1994; Sugirtharajah, 1994; Wright, 1994). Other women have remained within these religious groups, but have recognized or reconstructed their view of God to reflect feminine or feminist beliefs. Some women have become involved with the ancient religious practices associated with goddess worship, while others have developed a spiritual side without connection to any specific group (Hunt, 1995).

Reflection: Take time to reflect on your own experiences of organized religion and the influences of men and women within that religion.

Language

Recommendations have been made to change religious language to be inclusive, with names of God altered to be 'Mother' or 'Friend' (Hebblethwaite, 1984; Storkey, 1985; LaChance, 1991; Hunt, 1995). In Judaeo-Christian belief biblical passages have been explored and shown to demonstrate that God's image is referred to in feminine ways (Atkins, 1998). Such discovery may be a challenge to women with long-term belief, as they face the suggestion that God may be 'Mother' too. This may lead to conflict, as such thought does not fit generally into the common religious view of a male God, though the concept of a mother God may also be exclusive to some (King, 1993). Storkey (1985) points out the danger of reconstructing the image we have of God to such an extent that a new god is created just to meet our own needs. This may be solved through the concept of an androgynous 'Being', who is neither male nor female, but carries both masculine and feminine characteristics (Storkey, 1985; King, 1993). What this Being may be called is solved by King (1993) who consistently refers to an 'all-encompassing Ultimate Reality'.

In Catholicism the Virgin Mary is recognized as a role model or point of identity for women (Storkey, 1985; Schott and Henley, 1996), with some cultural groups personalizing her as 'our Mother' (Magana and Clark, 1995). Some women feel uncomfortable with this iconization of Jesus' mother, preferring the mother-worship of God, as highlighted. Storkey (1985) points out that Mary was only a woman. She was not God. Within other religious beliefs there may be more than one god or goddess with particular functions and characteristics (Holm and Bowker, 1994a; Schott and Henley, 1996). This implies that the problem with language may only be in religions where there is only a single God-figure worshipped.

Reflection: Do you think the use of non-inclusive language is a barrier to being involved in organized religion?

Transcendence through non-mainstream religions

For other groups of women, experience of transcendence is through eco-worship, the worship of nature or creative forces. This may be through worship of the earth, often called Mother Earth after Greek mythology

(Kahn, 1995), through the moon, the Moon Mother (Rich, 1992) or Mother Sea (King, 1993), with other deity names being the Great Mother, Mother Goddess or the Great Goddess (Achterberg, 1990; King, 1993; Kahn, 1995; Davis-Floyd and Davis, 1997). It is suggested that there was goddess worship prior to the advent of a male supreme being which was then actively suppressed (Achterberg, 1990; King, 1993; Kahn, 1995). The rise in feminism and greater female self-awareness has led to some returning to this ancient form of goddess worship, as a step of rejection of the more traditional religions (Rich, 1992; King, 1993).

Search for meaning and purpose

It is apparent from the definitions of spirituality explored that a search for a meaning and purpose for existence is a common aspect of men's and women's lives. This may be through the transcendent relationship with a god, as already described (Fish and Shelley, 1978; Labun, 1988; Burkhardt, 1994; Price et al., 1995), through work or creativity (Burnard, 1988; Labun, 1988), through relationships (King, 1993; Burkhardt, 1994; Price et al., 1995), through choices and actions (Burkhardt, 1994), or through political or social involvement (King, 1993; Kahn, 1995). Meaning may also be elicited through particular events, or through significant objects (Stanworth, 1997). Waugh (1992) also includes 'fulfilment in life', which would indicate that the search for a purpose has achieved some success. Within the 1990s searching for meaning may also be through achieving wholeness and health, as through mystical New Age philosophy, or through physical fitness and having the 'perfect body'. Women may specifically search for a meaning and purpose for themselves in the aspects of pregnancy and motherhood (Hebblethwaite, 1984; Rubin, 1984; Bergum, 1989; LaChance, 1991; Rich, 1992; Kahn, 1995; Hampton, 1995).

Reflection: Do you agree with the suggestion that most people are searching for meaning and purpose in life?

Humanism

For a person with belief, meaning may be found in religious practices. For those without belief, they must look for meaning in something other than God. Burnard (1988) describes the concept of 'secular humanism', where the person gains meaning for life from having responsibility for themselves and then developing responsibility for others. Stoll (1989, p. 7) expands the definition of humanism to state that '. . . the person has consciously or unconsciously chosen values that become the supreme focus of life and/or around which life is organized. These supreme values motivate people's lifestyle toward fulfilment of their goals, needs, and aspirations'.

Finding values by which to live is a significant aspect of human existence. Whereas those with a personal belief in God may find their values through religious rules or rituals, those without belief need to develop their values through assessment of knowledge and experience.

Women's meaning and purpose

Within modern society women may search to establish a role and be expected to fit in with social behavioural patterns in order to 'belong' and be accepted. For some women there is a desperate need to feel accepted in society, and the assumption is made that motherhood will fulfil this need (Harris, 1994). Further exploration of the implications of this will be explored in later chapters.

A sense of purpose for women may also be searched for within the socio-political framework of feminism. King (1993) writes that feminists are searching for 'wholeness and integration' and that this is what is at 'the heart of spirituality'. Within this context she says that it is not just a personal search, but one that leads to accepting responsibility socially and being politically active. This gives credence to Waugh's (1992) argument that there are two levels of spirituality, vertical and horizontal (see Chapter 1).

Women's search for meaning may lead to a new discovery of the feminine self, and be developed through integrating with other women. This discovery of self as part of spiritual awareness will be discussed later, but it is appropriate to record it as an element in women's search for meaning.

Reflection: From the text you have read is it right to suggest that women's searches for meaning are any different to those of men?

Belonging or connecting

Tucakovic (1994, p. 16) defines spirituality by saying it '. . . is the connection within our being, the connection to beings and the connection to other'. Belonging and connecting is also included in Lane's definition (Lane, 1987 cited in Harrison and Burnard, 1993, p. 11) as '. . . the desire to belong to someone, something, somewhere'.

Whereas the desire to belong appears to be more applicable to within groups, such as societal (Rubin, 1984; Bergum, 1989; Magana *et al.*, 1995), religious (Sered, 1991) or political (King, 1993; Kahn, 1995), connecting appears to be more on a personal, relationship level (Gaskin, 1977; LaChance, 1991; Burkhardt, 1994; Tucakovic, 1994; Hampton, 1995). It could be argued that the desire to belong is applicable to both genders, but it is not known to what extent the ability to develop connecting relationships may be more related to feminine aspects of spirituality. It is argued that the feminist tendency to highlight connection as being important suggests that women perceive that separations are present and need to be overcome (King, 1993).

Reflection: Do you believe women desire or form relationships in a different way to men? Does it matter if they do or don't?

Group belonging

Researchers have indicated the importance of clothing in women's ability to establish themselves in the social group in the western world (Rubin, 1984; Bergum, 1989). Certainly this may be applicable to men as well. How people dress, particularly as teenagers, demonstrates which group they aspire to belong to and may lead to acceptance by others within that group. Expectations of behaviour may also indicate group belonging. Different cultural groups may use rituals in order to recognize particular life stages and establish belonging within that society (Kitzinger, 1989; Davies, 1994; Holm and Bowker, 1994; Callister, 1995; Schott and Henley, 1996; Kitzinger, 1997; Yearley, 1997). A woman is expected to conform to local practices to belong socially, but this may also be a way of developing self-esteem through societal and self-acceptance (Goodenough, 1991). Belonging, in the social sense therefore, appears to require the woman to conform in order to receive acceptance into the group.

Reflection: To what extent do you believe this to be true? Is it true for men as well?

Religious belonging by women may also be accompanied by ritual and expectation (Sered, 1991; Holm and Bowker, 1994b; Callister, 1995; Magana and Clark, 1995; Schott and Henley, 1996). These issues will be further explored in the context of pregnancy and birth (see Chapter 3).

Political groupings may take many forms, and belonging may range from something as simple as accepting the principles behind the group, to active and proactive participation. Women may be particularly drawn to organizations involved in environmental improvement (Baginsky, 1986; La Chance, 1991; King, 1993), while others may develop interests in world or local peace initiatives (King 1993). Also the self-growth that may accompany a spiritual quest may lead to an embracing of feminism in one of its forms. King (1993) describes this in terms of 'sisterhood' and a 'relatedness' with all women, associating with all their experiences. It would suggest that belonging to one of these political groups would reflect a need to have a sense of purpose. However, such desire for involvement may not be isolated to women's experience of spirituality.

Spiritual connection

Spiritual 'connecting' may be regarded as more than just belonging to a particular group or social sphere. Burkhardt's (1994) research into the spiritual perspective of women identified connecting as a significant element. Though the research was limited to a particular area, the participants came from various religious, racial and ethnic groups and included those without religious belief, suggesting that the results could be applied to women generally. The study identified these women's connections with:

- History and the future
- God or 'Ultimate Other'
- Self
- Nature
- Others (Burkhardt, 1994, pp 18–19).

Some of these issues have already been discussed in relation to transcendence. The connection with experiences of women in history has been described by other writers as significant in pregnancy and birth (Gaskin, 1977; LaChance, 1991; Raphael-Leff, 1991; Rich, 1992; Rothman, 1994; Kahn, 1995; O'Shea, 1998). The need for women to have connecting relationships with others apart from family members appears from this study to be a specific aspect of feminine spirituality. This may be demonstrated through involvement in caring communities, such as church, or through caring relationships, either from being the carer or being cared for (Sered, 1991; Burkhardt, 1994; Magana and Clark, 1995).

Reflection: What are your thoughts about these suggestions concerning women's desire to form connecting relationships outside the family group? Is this true for every culture?

Relational aspects

Relationships generally have been explored through the context of belonging and connecting. However, also included in the definitions of spirituality are other aspects of relationship, such as giving and receiving love and giving to others through practical care (Dickinson, 1975; Fish and Shelley, 1978; Highfield and Cason, 1983; Lane, 1987; Labun, 1988; Waugh, 1992; Burkhardt, 1994). It has been suggested that a human relationship is needed by the spirit (Dickinson, 1975) and this may be something that is more enhanced in feminine spirituality (Dobbie, 1991). Others have suggested that spirituality is demonstrated through actions to others (Highfield and Cason, 1983; Waugh, 1992; Burkhardt, 1994). The giving of care will be explored in a later chapter within the context of midwifery care, but it is appropriate to mention that this is relevant to the woman in her role as a partner and mother, because of her loving and giving relationships within these contexts.

The Judaeo-Christian belief of unconditional love by God, and acceptance of that love, may give the woman a greater capacity to give love to others (Fish and Shelley, 1978). A humanistic approach will place value on other people, which may also increase the woman's ability to love (Burnard, 1988). It is not known if women who have been able to receive love from others are more able to give love, though Flagler and Nicoll (1990) suggest that women without a nurturing and supporting 'social environment' are not able to give in the same way as those who are supported.

Reflection: What are your reactions to the above suggestions about women's relationships and ability to love?

Self-development

The concept of 'self' has been identified as an element of spirituality, whether in terms of being able to make choices (Lane, 1987), in self-becoming (Dobbie, 1991; King, 1993; Burkhardt, 1994; Tucakovic, 1994), in having a sense of self-worth (Burkhardt, 1994; Price *et al.*, 1995) or in self-belief (Waugh, 1992). This concept is probably not an issue specifically or uniquely for women. It is argued that the effect of the questioning of gender identity by feminists is to search for a new female self (King, 1993). King goes on to suggest that this indicates the need for development of a 'new male self' and a subsequent change in relationship between the two groups. However, there may be particular areas or times in women's lives when such growth may occur. Dobbie's (1991) study, focussing upon the spiritual experience of a group of women at the time of 'mid-life transition', discovered that there were particular 'trigger events' when these women began to be more self-aware (she calls it 'interiority'). These were:

- Children leaving home.
- Changes in employment or taking up study.
- The end of a marital relationship.
- Physical changes through pregnancy or the menopause.
- Personal growth.

Reflection: What are your reactions to events such as these? Could this self-awareness be applied to men as well?

Childbearing has been identified as being a time of self-development in women's lives (Rubin, 1984; Belenky *et al.*, 1986). This implies that such life-changing events may be particular times when women undertake a period of self-growth that may lead to a development of spiritual consciousness.

This concept of self was also identified as learning to love oneself which led to a change in loving others. King (1993) also argues for women to love and affirm themselves because 'they are so often maimed and moulded by subjection, self-effacement and rejection'. This self-affirmation may grow out of what Eisenstein (1984) calls 'a sense of affiliation and connection with others, rather than in competition with them'. The quality of women's relationships is therefore seen as being valuable in the process of self-growth. Dobbie (1991) indicates that for the women in her study there was 'a shift in consciousness from self in relation to others to self in relation to self'. The issue that women may be constantly living their lives for and through other people may lead to a woman depriving herself of her spirituality until such a time when these relationships change or move on (King, 1993).

Women's concepts of selfhood may also be linked to their concepts of physical self (King, 1993). Feminist writers have argued for and against the value placed on women's bodily experiences, some seeing this as the 'root cause of woman's oppression and inferiority' (King, 1993) while others view the differences as something to be celebrated (Rhodes, 1997).

Reflection: What are your thoughts about the suggestion that women may be frequently living their lives through and for other people? Is this any different for men?

Hope and faith

Stoll (1979) states that 'To hope is to have a future'. This hope is recognized as a sign of spiritual well-being, an indication that having hope gives a sense of purpose to life (Highfield and Cason, 1983). Waugh (1992) indicates that hope can have a positive effect on healing and, in contrast, that death may be the result of 'hopelessness'.

In discussing spiritual care, Labun (1988) identifies hope as an action illustrating spiritual integrity. In another study hope was linked with 'potential' (O'Shea, 1998), which does give an image of something positive to which we may look forward. In human terms 'potential' may be seen in people, things or situations. This would suggest that positive attitudes and behaviours may be indicators of a spiritual life. It is unlikely that such attitudes are totally the province of women.

Reflection: Do you believe this last statement to be true?

Faith may be regarded as '. . . a belief in or assent to something that cannot be seen' (Carson, 1989b, p. 27) or, when used in context of relationship, it may be '. . . a way of acting and responding in relation to the other' (Carson, 1989b, p. 28).

Expression of faith does not need to be religious but could be related to other issues (Harrison and Burnard, 1993) such as:

- Career
- Country of origin
- Family life
- Money
- Self.

However, Waugh (1992, p. 24) argues that '. . . it is possible to have belief without faith, yet impossible to have faith without belief'.

Reflection: What are your responses to this statement?

She further indicates that faith is a result of belief becoming 'personal and meaningful' (Waugh, 1992). It is unlikely that faith is a spiritual element that is exclusive to women, although it is possible that the way it is expressed may be different (for instance, the use of creativity). These issues would benefit from further research.

Intuition

Though intuitive behaviour has not been recognized as a specific element of spirituality, it has been identified in relation to spiritual care (Gaskin, 1977; Waugh, 1992; Harrison and Burnard, 1993; Davis-Floyd and Davis, 1997). It has also been suggested to be a particularly feminine characteristic (Estes, 1992; Burkhardt, 1994; Davis-Floyd and Davis, 1997).

Reflection: What is your response to the suggestion that intuition is a particularly feminine trait?

Various characteristics of intuition have been identified (Bastick, 1982 quoted in Davis-Floyd and Davis, 1997) and include:

- Sudden and immediate awareness of knowing.
- Association of affect with insight.
- Non-analytical, non-rational and non-logical nature of experience.
- Empathy.
- Creativity.
- Certainty of truth in the insights.

Rew (1989, p. 56) defines intuition as '. . . a way of knowing that bypasses our usual reliance on logic and linear analysis'. In our high technology society, this form of knowledge may be regarded as less valuable because of not being scientific, whereas in more traditional societies intuitive thought and knowledge is more highly valued (Belenky *et al.*, 1986). However, Estes (1992, p. 10) suggests that, if women are not in touch with their instinct, they are living in 'a semi-destroyed state and images and powers that are natural to the feminine are not allowed full development'. This would imply that all women who live in technological societies and are not instinctive in their behaviour are not complete!

Reflection: How would you respond to Estes' statement?

It is suggested that the development of intuition is better in situations where women are in groups together, as there is less competition with other ways of knowing or not open to condemnation by those with logical reasoning processes (Davis, 1995). Such argument does imply that women are not capable of logical thought and would use intuition in favour of reasoning. Conversely, it implies that all men use logical reasoning and are unable to be intuitive. Such an argument cannot be accepted without investigating male groups to discover how intuitive reasoning develops among them or how women also use logical reasoning.

Story-telling

The telling of stories may be an integral part of feminine spirituality. But is story-telling only applicable to women, as in many religions stories are used to provide messages and give guidance to followers, and were usually told by men? Exploration of the use of language and the specific use of metaphoric phrases as indicators of spirituality has suggested that this is not limited to women (Stanworth, 1997). It could be asked, too, whether the demonstration of spirituality is in the telling of descriptive stories, as in those suggested by Estes (1992), or in the woman telling her own personal story? Both Burkhardt (1998) and Taylor (1997) have described the telling in respect of the person's own life. This telling has been suggested (Burkhardt, 1998) to reveal:

- The connections that give support.
- The relationships needing healing.
- The sources of the person's strength.
- The experiences that have given meaning to the person's life so far.
- The questions the person has in respect of life's meaning.

Taylor (1997) states that people tell stories to:

- Allow the person to order and connect aspects of life experiences.
- Enable organization of experience and thoughts.
- Allow reflection and observation.
- Make sense of the story.
- Enable connection and intimacy with others.
- Leave a 'legacy' for others.
- Relate 'values, beliefs and interpretations' of life.

Kirkham (1997) suggests that being able to relate and establish our personal stories enables us to understand and give meaning to the experiences.

For the story to make a difference it would seem appropriate to expect that the teller needs someone to tell the story to, someone who is prepared to listen. For King (1993) the 'feminist consciousness raising' between groups of women, to enable understanding of each other's situation, is linked to telling and listening to each other's story. Story-telling being linked with feminine spirituality in this way may be as a result of women:

- Being more willing to share with others.
- Being better at listening to others.
- Having more time to spend meeting with other women.
- Being more able to interpret meaning from the relating of stories.

As with the other spiritual issues mentioned, it will take further research to establish if story-telling can be described completely as an attribute of feminine spirituality.

> *Reflection: Do you think story-telling in this sense is limited to women? Do you think it meets a spiritual need or a physical or emotional need?*

Conclusion

From the above information it can be supposed that there is no clear definition of the attributes of spirituality that are particularly feminine in nature. As suggested at the beginning of the chapter, each person, whether male or female, has both masculine and feminine characteristics that will be enhanced or suppressed in different situations and according to personality. It would be necessary to perform much more research to demonstrate these character differences, but even then it would be difficult to differentiate between the sexes. From this it is suggested that, in issues of spirituality, each person should be treated individually and their needs and aspirations addressed accordingly, as opposed to being given the labels of male or female. This is a true aim of giving holistic care and is also the aim of 'women-centred' care in midwifery. Within the following chapter these issues of spirituality are enlarged and discussed in relation to pregnancy and childbirth.

Transcendence and hope and the valuing midwife

Transcendence

The experience of transcendence for a pregnant woman will reflect that of women in general, as described in Chapter 2. It may involve a relationship with a Higher Being, in or out of an organized religion or may involve personal aspirations to increased self-knowledge.

Religious belief

For those involved in religious groups, the birth of a child is often a time when specific rituals take place in order to welcome his or her arrival. These may involve just the close family or the whole company of believers. In many cultures specific ceremonies take place at the birth of a child as it is regarded as a 'rite of passage' for both the new mother and the baby. Thus birth is regarded as a significant time, a time of transformation both in the sociological sense and spiritually.

For the pregnant woman with faith a transcending relationship with a Higher Being may already be a very real aspect of her spiritual self. Hebblethwaite's (1984) description of her experiences of motherhood and beliefs reflects a growth of relationship with God (whom she always refers to as 'she') during pregnancy, birth and in the postnatal period while caring for three small children. Pregnancy and motherhood may lead some women to discover the feminine aspects of God (LaChance, 1991) which challenge women with long-term belief, and may lead to conflict, as such thought does not fit into the common Judaeo-Christian or Muslim view of a male expression of God.

The Virgin Mary

The Catholic expression of the Christian faith has created a role model for women in the elevation of the Virgin Mary (Storkey, 1985; Schott and Henley, 1996), with some cultures personalizing her as 'our Mother' (Magana and Clark, 1995). It is suggested that this personalization provides a 'coping mechanism' which may ultimately provide a protective effect to women with belief and to their babies (Magana and Clark, 1995). The possible reasons for this are given as:

- Those who have religious belief will tend to follow more positive health behaviour patterns, which may subsequently lead to better health in pregnancy and improved birth outcomes.
- Faith gives the women higher self-esteem, gives meaning to life and involves them in practices that bring 'cultural richness' to their lives.
- Prayer may have a place in good health. The church may be a place of peace in an otherwise stressful life.
- Church life provides an extended network of women with similar values, providing teaching and support.

Though this supposition is related to one culture, these factors may also be applicable to any who have strong religious belief and who are active within a community of believers. A large study of Australian women, comparing religious values and practices and pregnancy outcomes, demonstrated that those who had greater religious commitment had better pregnancy outcomes (Najman *et al.*, 1988). They suggest this may be attributable to the woman's lifestyle and healthy behaviour patterns. However, they also suggest it would be difficult to encourage adjustment of these women's lifestyle behaviours in pregnancy without dealing with their underlying values and beliefs.

Growth of belief

Pregnancy and birth have frequently been described as a journey or a rite of passage, a time of significant growth for the woman. For the woman with belief, the time may also include a growth in relationship with her god, with a desire to increase the activities associated with her particular religion, such as prayer, reading or attendance of religious meetings. The relationship is described through the acknowledgement of the Higher Being as Creator (Hebblethwaite, 1984) and the 'miraculous' nature of the experience (Gaskin, 1977; Rubin, 1984; Sered, 1991; Hernes, 1996).

Positive pain

It has been suggested in Christian belief that the vulnerability of the woman during birth may lead to an openness to an increased experience of God's power, strength and love, and the pain of childbirth has been viewed as positive and may encourage greater closeness to God. Rich (1992) also relates to inescapable pain as being something 'useable' that can lead 'beyond the limits of the experience itself'. Women in Lundgren and Dahlberg's (1998) study also viewed the pain positively by suggesting that it brought them closer to the baby or gave them strength to cope with 'the new demands' of being a mother. However, it is not known if this is just significant for those who have a strong belief prior to pregnancy, or whether it includes those who have minimal or no belief.

A midwife interviewed in research, describing the religious experience of some Jewish women during pregnancy and birth, stated that women who had pregnancy difficulties turned to God for help. She suggested that when the birth was normal the women viewed the experience more as a personal challenge as opposed to reliance on God. When things went wrong, however, they turned to God for help (Sered, 1991). The indication from this is that, if birth progresses normally, without undue stress to the woman, she will go through the event without reference to God, and it is only if there are problems that she will turn for outside help. It is not known if this is applicable to those with strong beliefs in other religions. In O'Shea's (1998) recent small study, religious belief was viewed as a 'source of reassurance and consolation' for the women, especially when it was suggested that a baby may experience problems when born. It is suggested that spiritual distress may bring a person into a deeper relationship with God (Smucker, 1996), and therefore it may follow that a distressing pregnancy or birth could do the same for the woman involved (Brown, 1993). Some who have experienced termination (Marck, 1994) or the birth of a handicapped child (Diachuk, 1994) have described turning to God to help them through the experience.

Expression of spirituality

For the women in Sered's (1991) study, the researcher concluded that they did not regard their birth experiences as 'peak incidents' in their lives, or as particularly religiously significant, but more as another incident among many during 'the continuum of life and relationship'. This study is limited by the subjects all being of the Jewish faith, where the men tend to undertake the majority of the rituals and prayers associated with the birth of the child. The researcher suggested their culture, where Jewish law regards birth as 'polluting', denied the women a language to express the spirituality of the experience. For women of other beliefs or cultures, where they experience a sacredness in birth, the ability to express spirituality may be different (Balin, 1988; Sokoloski, 1995; Callister et al., 1996; Morgan, 1996; Khalaf and Callister, 1997). Rubin's (1984) larger, cross-cultural study of maternal experience led her to conclude (p. 129): 'There is an increased orienting toward and conviction in the omniscience and control of a Creator. Signs, omens, dream images, and the experience of others are not ignored. Wishes are replaced with prayers.' This would indicate that an awareness of a higher being or power may not be limited to those with belief. However, this is not conclusive without information regarding the subject's personal beliefs prior to pregnancy.

Reflection: In what spiritual ways have women you know with beliefs prior to pregnancy coped with pregnancy and labour? Have you known women change their beliefs because of bad experiences?

Antenatal issues

Belief in a Higher Being may be of varying degrees, ranging from a belief of something else being there to an active participation in a relationship, often, but not always, accompanied by involvement in religious activities. The levels of belief may be significant in how a woman approaches some of the aspects of pregnancy and birth. For instance, some women may find the idea of antenatal testing for fetal abnormality abhorrent, as they are prepared to accept 'God's will' for their life and the life of their child (Rothman, 1994). This may be carried to an extreme limit, where a couple's belief in God prevents them from accepting medical care, with the result that the baby may not live or be damaged. Such reactions will be a challenge to the couple's carers (see Box 1).

Case history 1

Ellie, a 43-year-old woman with two teenage children, discovers she is pregnant when she attends her GP for unexplained amenorrhoea. She is quite shocked and the GP recommends that she attends the hospital for an ultrasound scan to assess dating of the pregnancy and outlines the antenatal screening tests for fetal abnormality with her. Ellie decides not to have this performed immediately but to go home and discuss it with her husband. Together they decide to approach their religious leader, as they have a strong faith. After some time of counsel with him they decide to have the ultrasound scan but to decline the screening blood test, as they feel they would not have a termination of the pregnancy should something be discovered. The next day Clare, the community midwife attached to the surgery, makes contact with Ellie to make a booking appointment. Ellie tells her she wishes to decline the antenatal testing, and Clare indicates to her that she supports her choice.

During the next week, Ellie and her husband attend the local hospital antenatal clinic for the ultrasound appointment. Having estimated the age of the fetus as 11 weeks the radiographer measures the nuchal-translucency thickness without saying anything to the couple about what she is doing (Snijders *et al.*, 1998). In the interview with the obstetrician afterwards he recommends for her to have screening tests performed as he suspects the presence of Down's syndrome. As a couple they refuse again, but the doctor tries to pressure them to do so, enlisting the help of the clinic Sister. The couple still decline and leave the clinic feeling upset by the experience. Clare is contacted by the Sister to ask for her assistance in persuading the couple. Clare expresses her support of the couple's decision but agrees to visit Ellie. During the visit Clare listens carefully to Ellie's views and gives her balanced information on the risks involved with Down's syndrome diagnosis. Ellie still declines testing and goes ahead with the pregnancy with Clare's support, and the continued support of her religious leader.

Eventually she gives birth to a healthy, term baby girl in hospital, thankful that she had not gone ahead with any further tests.

For other women their belief may allow them antenatal testing, to discover if there is abnormality present, but only in order to prepare themselves for the situation prior to birth, and not to accept termination of the pregnancy. Societal attitudes towards termination are closely related to religious belief (Illsley and Hall, 1976; Wikman *et al.,* 1992), and the potential termination of a child remains a sensitive issue, whether the woman expresses a belief in a personal God or not.

The emotional and physical changes of pregnancy may cause a woman to evaluate her belief. Pregnancy may highlight issues from her upbringing in a family with religious affiliation and lead her to question specific rules related to pregnancy. Pregnancy often creates stronger family bonds, with greater involvement and influence by the woman's mother (Raphael-Leff, 1991; Schott and Henley, 1996). Conflict may arise within families where the woman decides not to adhere to the family convictions. Her ability to form or maintain a transcendent relationship may thus be prevented.

Reflection: Are you aware of women who have questioned your or others' care because of their beliefs?

Labour aspects

Belief may also be significant in the way a woman makes decisions regarding her care for labour. Complete denial of all medical intervention is unusual, but others may express their belief through wanting a birth in the home environment, to allow God's will to take place or to enable them to practise religious rituals. It has been argued that it may be impossible to have a spiritual experience of birth in a hospital environment (Kahn, 1995). However, Stockley (1986) suggests that this can be facilitated through the couple 'preparing' the labour room spiritually when they enter, or by the use of 'absent visualization' methods if they have visited the hospital prior to birth.

Women may also express belief through denial of pain relief or refusing induction of labour, as this will interfere with 'God's timing', or through refusal of caesarean section and blood transfusion (Schott and Henley, 1996).

Case history 2

Reported in a paper in *Health Matters* (Stone, 1993) is the court case of a woman, S. In this case she was admitted to hospital in spontaneous labour. She had ruptured membranes for 6 days and was over her due date. The baby was thought to be dying but S refused a caesarean section on strong religious grounds. The hospital was granted permission to perform a caesarean despite her refusal. The baby died and S survived.

Those associated with particular religions may wish to practise ceremonies related to labour. In Sered's (1991) study, the couple tended to perform these prior to going to the hospital, which indicates the problems associated with accepting personal practices, even in an overtly religious society such as Israel. Within our society the use of ceremony to express belief, and rituals, including chanting, music, prayer, use of candles, care over personal hygiene or ritual hand washing, may all be denied to women giving birth in a hospital setting. In situations of perinatal loss, awareness of religious rituals involving death are important and will need to be explored with each couple involved (Brown, 1993; Schott and Henley, 1996).

> *Reflection: How would you react as a carer if a woman chose to refuse midwifery or medical intervention on religious grounds? How would you feel if she or the baby were subsequently damaged as a result of this belief? How may support be given to those wishing to practice religious rituals?*

Transcendence without God

Transcendence may not mean a relationship with a Higher Being, but a greater desire for self-knowledge (Lane, 1987). This may be expressed by pregnant women in different forms. The development of a new life may be regarded as the ultimate act of creativity, and therefore it may not be unusual for pregnant women to have desires to be more in touch with nature. This may be through a desire to be near the sea (Kahn, 1995), or through being aware of the life cycles of the earth and ecology (LaChance,

1991; Parvati Baker, 1993; Rawlings, 1995). Others may experience a greater desire to be creative themselves, such as through artistic expression, poetry, making things or gardening.

This link to nature has been connected to the way the will no longer controls the body during labour, and the ability for the woman to be able to breastfeed her baby, in line with other mammals (Kahn, 1995). Estes (1992) suggests too that women may become in touch with a 'wild' self during pregnancy, comparing women's behaviour with that of a wolf. The recent interest in labouring and giving birth in water may be related to the desire to be associated with nature (Cohen, 1996), though the use of water for relaxation and pain relief also meets the physical needs of the woman (Odent, 1984).

The connection of the pregnant woman with the earth may not be surprising, with the associated links of planting seeds and giving birth to new life. Often earth is called Mother Earth, after Greek mythology (Kahn, 1995), and women who are regarded as very motherly are called 'earth mothers'. As highlighted in the previous chapter, women may express nature worship in other ways, including through goddess worship (Achterberg, 1990; King, 1993; Kahn, 1995). A pregnant woman's involvement with forms of alternative worship may lead to rejection of traditional forms of care, and a wish to experience birth in alternative settings (Hillyer, 1987). Alternatively, pregnancy may lead to a quest for understanding in a more feminine belief structure (Kahn, 1995).

Pregnancy and birth bring change to women and their lives. The creative nature of the experience may lead to a greater awareness of 'something beyond' the earthly realms, as well as becoming more in touch with her femininity. It is recognized that women will view childbirth as 'creation' and it is suggested that participation in the experience makes us all 'co-creators' (O'Shea, 1998). The issue of transcendence will need to be explored further, in the light of Rubin's (1984) research into maternal experience, to assess if her supposition of an increased belief in God is true for those of all beliefs or no belief.

Reflection: Have women you have known demonstrated increased interest in the natural world or creativity during pregnancy?

Hope and faith

For pregnant women hope may be a significant element of spirituality. There is hope:

● For a live, well baby (Rubin, 1984).
● To be able to cope with labour and mothering (LaChance, 1991).

- For a natural labour (LaChance, 1991).
- For a safe birth (Rubin, 1984).
- To be a good parent (Hebblethwaite, 1984; Berryman and Windridge, 1995).

Hebblethwaite (1984) also describes the hope of producing future generations through her children, and leaving a 'lasting mark' on humanity. For the women of O'Shea's (1998) study, hope was viewed in relation to the 'potential' of the baby, not only for the future of the family but also for the future of humanity.

Reflection: Have you been aware of any of these 'hopes' in pregnant women?

The opposite emotion to hope could be regarded as fear, which is identified as a real experience for many, if not all, pregnant women at some time (Hebblethwaite, 1984; Rubin, 1984; Marck, 1994; McGeary, 1994; Kahn, 1995; Sherr, 1995). For women in Sered's (1991) study, feelings of needing to protect their babies resulted in ritualistic behaviour. Fear is thus transformed into action. McGeary's (1994) study of 'guarding' in women who were experiencing high risk pregnancies identified a point, termed 'reaching a safe stage', where the women were able to transfer from feelings of fear to one of hope. It has been highlighted that though professionals are quick to give information about and use technology, the same enthusiasm and time is not given to dealing with the woman's hopes and fears, which, it is suggested, shows a lack of value placed on these feelings and the care required (Marck *et al.*, 1994). It seems apparent that for a woman to have a spiritual experience she will need to transfer from feelings of fear to one of hope, and to do this she may need the support of understanding caregivers.

The consequence of faith and religious belief have been discussed in the section on transcendence. However, women may have a spiritual experience through faith in her own body to achieve a natural birth, or through faith in the carers to meet her needs. The experience may also be through the depth of relationship with her partner and the belief in the power of that support. Her surroundings at the time may also be a factor in her ability to achieve a spiritual experience. Failure in any of these situations to meet her beliefs may result in distress, due to not having achieved her spiritual goal.

Reflection: In what ways may women's hopes and fears be addressed and supported? Has the behaviour of women you know been influenced by their fears? In what ways has a pregnant woman's faith influenced her actions?

The midwife who values and accepts

The ability to recognize the worth of the individual appears to be a common theme in papers relating to spiritual care. This recognition could be demonstrated through:

- Giving intense care and respect (Price *et al.*, 1995).
- Being non-judgemental (Dickinson, 1975).
- Respect and understanding of the person's beliefs and customs despite them being different to those of the carer (Labun, 1988; Davis-Floyd and Davis, 1997).

In midwifery terms, Gaskin (1977) writes that it is expected of a spiritual midwife to love everyone in her care in the same way. This indicates that each woman should be treated as an individual, and her cultural needs recognized and met (Schott and Henley, 1996; Callister *et al.*, 1996; Morgan, 1996; Khalaf and Callister, 1997). However, there are indications that impressions of people are developed over time, and that first encounters result in stereotyping (Hicks, 1993). Research has noted that information and communication by midwives to women of lower social groups tends to be inferior to that given to those in higher groups (Kirkham, 1989; Hunt and Symonds, 1995). Also, the facial and bodily appearance of the person results in differing perceptions (Hicks, 1993; Hunt and Symonds, 1995). Midwives may also be in need themselves, and may treat those women who are unconsciously meeting those needs in a different way (Clarke, 1996). The implication is that women may not be treated with equal respect and value as people, but that value is placed on other issues.

Reflection: Do you believe it is possible to treat each person individually while still meeting the needs of the carer?

Valuing through continuity of care

The women in Berg *et al.*'s (1996) phenomenological study of their encounters with midwives indicated the need to be respected and treated as equals. The researchers conclude that this need to be recognized as an individual is met by the woman being affirmed and by being familiar with the midwife and by her environment. This familiarity through providing continuity of carer has other benefits, such as:

- Giving the woman confidence.
- Increasing feelings of self-worth.

• Increasing the woman's feelings of power and control (Belbin, 1996; Page, 1996).

However, the midwife needs to have attributes of caring (Halldorsdottir *et al.*, 1996). The woman being in control of decision-making increases her power, and this can be achieved through being fully informed. In contrast, lack of information has been demonstrated to disempower women in labour (McKay, 1991), and uncaring attitudes and lack of respect lead to discouragement and a negative experience of childbirth (Halldorsdottir *et al.*, 1996). A study of women's experiences of complicated births showed the need for women to be valued and affirmed by their carers (Berg and Dahlberg, 1998). In situations where this occurred, the women were more likely to feel acceptance into their new role as mother, even if it was a highly technological experience. The authors state that this affirmation is not praise or agreeing with the person, but comes through viewing what the other person says as being significant and valid.

Reflection: In what ways may valuing another person enhance their experiences?

Giving value to stories

Burkhardt (1994) recommends that carers listen to a woman's story, thus placing value on who she is and what she has experienced. During the postnatal period it has been suggested that story-telling '. . . may also be cathartic at a deeper level for the woman' (Smith and Mitchell, 1996), which indicates that reliving events may meet a spiritual need in some women, as they feel their experience is valued by someone.

Effect of organization

In recent years it has been suggested that the institutional nature and impersonal structure of maternity care can make women feel devalued. It is further intimated that the use of birth protocols and needing to stick to them means women are not treated as individuals and that their creativity is disabled (Rawlings, 1995). In this way, the author continues, a woman's unique ability to give birth is restricted. It may thus be that true spiritual midwifery care will not be possible without the structure changing to have women's needs central to that care (Department of Health, 1993; Lovell, 1996; Page, 1996).

Reflection: Is it possible to give spiritual care despite the restraints of the present organization?

Conclusion

In summary, the element of transcendence for women may involve a relationship with a Higher Being, and may or may not be involved in a religious belief structure. For those with a religious belief, pregnancy and birth may involve:

- Significant rituals antenatally or in labour.
- Growth or conflict with her beliefs.
- Increase in activities surrounding her beliefs.
- Questioning of the care that is offered to her.

Alternatively, for other women pregnancy and birth may lead to:

- Self-growth.
- Wanting to be more close to nature.
- Being more artistically creative.
- Wanting to be more in touch with feminine issues.

The elements of hope and faith will be real for many women, as will the contrasting fears that may accompany pregnancy.

To provide support for these women the midwife needs to:

- Treat each person as valued, including accepting what the woman believes in.
- Aim to give continuity of care to enable giving value to the woman.
- Listen carefully to what women say and accept what they say.

4 *Searching for meaning and purpose and the enabling midwife*

The search for meaning and purpose in life appears to be an integral part of a person's spiritual experience (see previous chapters). The meanings of childbirth may be influenced by a number of personal issues, such as:

- Culture
- Age
- Parity
- Personal experience
- Religious faith or spiritual beliefs (see Nichols, 1996).

For a woman, pregnancy and motherhood may be a time when she specifically looks for or finds personal significance, and may be an important aspect of her maternal spiritual experience (Hebblethwaite, 1984; Rubin, 1984; Bergum, 1989; LaChance, 1991; Rich, 1992; Kahn, 1995; Hampton, 1995; Nichols, 1996; O'Shea, 1998). For those women unfortunate enough to experience perinatal loss, their search for meaning may be through developing an understanding of and purpose for the loss (Brown, 1993).

A woman entering pregnancy with belief in a Higher Being will weigh up the decisions and consequences of pregnancy in the light of the values she has already attained through that belief. She will find purpose through her experiences because of belief in 'God's will' or a plan for her life. As has already been indicated in the previous chapter in the section about transcendence, this may lead her to refuse or question medical or midwifery decisions that do not fit in with her concept of God's plan.

Choosing pregnancy

The desire for pregnancy and the decision to have a child may in itself be a search for meaning or, as Bergum (1989) called it, 'searching for life' through having a child. Flagler and Nicolls (1990) suggest that the meaning in pregnancy will be affected by the circumstances of the pregnancy. For some women pregnancy could be an active decision to 'create' and for others an unexpected event. The research into unexpected pregnancy showed a need for these women to search for a place in her self, or her life, for the child (Marck, 1994). A woman who has made an active decision to have a child may have commenced this process, and yet the fact that pregnancy is called a 'journey' indicates that the process of development is ongoing.

Pregnancy and motherhood

For some the quest for meaning begins with pregnancy. Rubin's (1984) research into maternal identity and experience suggests that the pregnant woman seeks:

- Physical safe passage.
- Acceptance of the child by the family.
- Acceptance of self and commitment as mother.
- 'Binding-in' to the child, by which Rubin means that the woman is exploring 'the meaning of giving, particularly the giving of self on behalf of another'.

Rubin continues by suggesting that a particular attribute of maternal conduct is looking for models to follow in pregnancy. This may be through:

- Discussions with members of her peer group who have already experienced pregnancy.
- Observation.
- Reading literature.
- Her own mother.
- The professionals with whom she is in contact.

Rubin suggests there is deliberate 'mimicry' and 'replication' of other women going through the same experience, or of professionals. Socio-logically in western society it is suggested that a woman will only be accepted as 'normal' or 'feminine' when she becomes a mother and that it is supposed to be a woman's 'destiny and role in life' (Gittens, 1985; Richardson, 1993). The implication is that the woman is searching to establish a role in society and fit in with the social behavioural patterns in order to 'belong' and be accepted. It is assumed by many that motherhood will fulfil this need for acceptance (Harris, 1994).

Reflection: How do you feel about the above observations regarding the acceptance of women in our western society being related to motherhood?

Richardson continues by suggesting that children give purpose and 'a reason for being'. This 'reason for being' gives women a sense of value –

an issue that has been identified by Wikman *et al.*'s (1992) research into attitudes of women towards aspects of reproduction in their society. Discovering a meaning for existence in motherhood may certainly be appropriate for some women. However, it may be more commonplace for motherhood to begin the process of searching. Research into women's development has shown that: 'Many women . . . experience giving birth to their children as a major turning point in their lives . . . In response to our question, "what was the most important learning experience you have ever had?" many mothers selected childbirth' (Belenky *et al.*, 1986, p. 35). Thus, the emotionally transforming time of childbirth may lead women into a process of questioning the meaning and purpose for their life.

Reflection: Do you believe women find a sense of purpose through childbirth?

Case history 3

Gloria was working as a health visitor when she became pregnant for the first time. She realized quite early in the pregnancy that she was not going to be able to continue working, as her partner worked long hours and they had no family close by to help with the child care. Though she was delighted with the pregnancy she found the thought of not having something to do a daunting prospect. She felt upset at not being able to *be* someone in society. When she eventually left work she shared some of her frustrations with her midwife, who suggested that Gloria needed to give herself time to focus her mind on having the baby and giving attention to her own needs. Gloria accepted this and spent the rest of the pregnancy trying to look after herself and getting to know the growing baby inside her. She attended a local parenthood and exercise class and began to get to know some of the women who lived locally. She began to discover that some of them were very needy, despite it being an affluent area, and that some of them had real anxieties about being mothers. After the birth the group met together for a reunion. It was here that Gloria discovered that she had a lot to offer to the group from her professional experience and suggested they may like to continue meeting regularly for postnatal support. She took an active leadership role, and through the links made was able provide support and guidance to those who wanted help. She also became involved in the local toddlers group and was frequently asked for advice. Gloria has been able to say that by letting go of her own aspirations and looking for her own needs to be met, she has found a sense of value in helping to meet the needs of the local women in her community.

In O'Shea's (1998) study, the participants indicated that their search for meaning was in some way focussed on the baby, and that the baby had fulfilled some kind of plan that was outside of their control – it 'was meant to be'. Others have identified this plan as being 'God's will' (Sokoloski, 1995; Khalaf and Callister, 1997). This fulfilment of a personal destiny may be a reality for a number of pregnant women and it is possible that such pregnancies may have resulted from an erratic use of contraception 'to see what happens'.

Trying to find meaning and purpose in pregnancy and birth may therefore be a process common to many women. It has been suggested that being able to find meaning in an experience will lead to 'coping and resolution' (Price *et al.*, 1995). Should a woman thus find meaning, purpose and fulfilment through the experience of childbirth, it could be assumed that her ability to cope with the stresses of motherhood will be improved.

Reflection: Do you agree with the supposition above that women who have found some fulfilment in the experience of childbirth cope better with motherhood?

The enabling midwife

An element of spiritual care identified is a willingness to help others find their own spiritual meaning in a situation. This may be through:

- Helping the person actively work through a situation (Dickinson, 1975).
- Establishing a relationship that aids communication of the client's needs (Labun, 1988).
- Affirmation and respect (Price *et al.*, 1995).
- Acknowledging when clients express 'feelings of meaninglessness' or demonstrate 'lack of purpose' (Harrison and Burnard, 1993).

In feminine terms, Burkhardt (1994) specifies that carers should be willing to assess how the woman extracts meaning from her life's events and discover what experiences have been easy or difficult for her.

Reflection: How may midwives help women find meaning in their experiences?

For midwives, this indicates a need to improve antenatal and postnatal assessments, to aid the communication process regarding spiritual issues. However, the midwife needs to be *willing* to help others, which indicates a need for a positive attitude towards providing spiritual care. It is to be remembered that the search for meaning may not be linked to religiosity, and that exploration may be required with respect to other sources, such as work (Burnard, 1988), relationships (King, 1993; Burkhardt, 1994; Price *et al.*, 1995) or politics and social issues (King, 1993; Kahn, 1995).

Reflection: Is it appropriate to expect a midwife to help women explore these issues?

Meaning from the birth experience

For some women meaning may be being searched for within the birth experience. This search may be facilitated through enabling the woman to be in control of the experience as much as possible, by giving her the space to make choices for herself (Page, 1993). A birth plan may be written evidence of the elements of the woman's search within the birthing process, and could be used as a trigger for discussion.

Reflection: In what way may a birth plan be used to trigger a discussion about the meanings of the experience to the woman?

Postnatal searching

Rawlings (1995) actively encourages a search for meaning through postnatal workshops that invite the women to discuss childbirth without reference to medical terms. She suggests that the sessions can provide freedom and healing for the bad memories. It could be argued that such workshops would not be necessary postnatally if women had been encouraged and facilitated to develop their search for meaning within the antenatal and labour periods.

Reflection: In what other ways may midwives encourage understanding of experiences and facilitate a woman's search for meanings?

Conclusion

This chapter has highlighted that a search for meaning and purpose in the events surrounding pregnancy and birth may be apparent for many women, and may therefore be evidence of their spirituality. A woman may search for meaning in:

● Becoming pregnant.
● Being pregnant.

- Motherhood.
- The baby.

The midwife may provide support to a woman searching for meaning by:

- Appropriate assessment of need.
- Having a positive attitude towards spiritual care and searching for meaning.
- Helping women work through issues in their personal situation.
- Developing a trusting and trustworthy relationship.
- Giving respect.
- Enabling the woman to be in control of her experience.
- Postnatal workshops.

5 *Connecting relationships and the midwife with presence*

Belonging or connecting

As highlighted in the previous chapter, belonging and connection are aspects of spirituality that may be specifically relevant to women. One may suppose that they will also be applicable to the pregnant woman.

Social grouping

For the pregnant woman the desire may be to belong to a social group labelled 'mothers'. Rubin's (1984) study showed that women tend to move from one social group to another that will be less effort to them because of the sharing of common experiences. The importance of the use of clothing to establish belonging in a social group is significant to pregnant women. This may be expressed through starting to wear clothes that show their pregnant state very early, although others may try and hide the fact for as long as possible, wanting to remain in the 'non-pregnant' group (Rubin, 1984; Bergum, 1989). All cultural groups use rituals in order to recognize the woman's pregnancy or her passage into motherhood. Social acceptance of the woman may be through her conforming to local practices, and acknowledgement by others of her changing state may assist in the woman's acceptance of her new self. This belonging may lead to raised self-esteem (Goodenough and Barratt, 1991). Consequently, the loss of a baby unexpectedly may lead to loss of self-esteem and to feelings of failure (Brown, 1993).

The indication is that the pregnant woman will wish for involvement in a group where she is made to feel valued. The friendships made in the antenatal period within new social groups will often become the main links socially in the postnatal period, especially in first pregnancies. In order to conform to the common goals for birth, the expectation may be for her to attend particular types of childbirth classes or to wish for certain forms of professional care.

Reflection: In what ways have you noticed women establishing a social identity during pregnancy?

45

Religious grouping

If pregnant women are to truly belong to religious groups, they may need to undertake certain rituals or ceremonies. In a study of Jewish women it was found that the ritual practices for birth were often undertaken in private, prior to entry into hospital, and many found it hard to maintain the expected religious practices during labour (Sered, 1991). Though these women came from a religious society, this study showed that most of them felt that the religious practices were not relevant to their experiences of childbirth.

Religious groups may have particular expectations of the way pregnant women should behave in relation to certain obstetric practices. Religious expectation may also be in conflict with the values of the society in which the woman is living. Her decision to accept or reject these practices may lead to guilt or a sense of failure, if she does not live up to the expectations. As already explored, a woman's experience of a relationship with her God may change in pregnancy or as a result of birth, leading to a resulting conflict with her desires to conform to the practices and beliefs of her religious group. Through involvement in religion, women may find a meaning and purpose for themselves and for having a new child.

Reflection: In what ways have you noticed the influence of religious groups upon the decisions or experiences of a pregnant woman?

Political grouping

Women's involvement in political activities during pregnancy may be through participation in groups such as the National Childbirth Trust or the Association for Improvements in the Maternity Services (AIMS), and their activities in standing for women's rights (Beech, 1986). Others may recognize a need to become involved in organizations motivated towards improving the environment or world peace, for the sake of the future of their new child (Baginsky, 1986; La Chance, 1991; Rhodes, 1997). Having contact with more women than men in pregnancy and after may lead to adopting a feminist viewpoint (Rich, 1992; Kahn, 1995). Such political involvement would imply the need to find a meaning in the pregnancy through achieving something positive for others.

Reflection: In what ways have you noticed women's political involvement in pregnancy and how has this been stimulated?

Connecting relationships

As described in the previous chapter, spiritual 'connecting' implies more than just belonging to a group. Based on Burkhardt's (1994) research into the spiritual perspective of women, the previous chapter identified the ways women develop connecting relationships. This may be transferred to the experiences of the pregnant woman.

Connecting with history

The significance of connecting with experiences of women in history during pregnancy and birth has been described by a number of writers (Gaskin, 1977; LaChance, 1991; Raphael-Leff, 1991; Rich, 1992; Rothman, 1994; Kahn, 1995; O'Shea, 1998). After a positive birth experience at home, LaChance (1991) writes of a 'reconnecting to the ancient power of birthing'. She continues by describing how the connection with her new daughter has enabled her to value her own mother for giving birth, and her grandmother and 'generations of women before me' (p. 13). Carolyn, a mother going through birth at The Farm community, described an experience during her labour of a telepathic relationship with all mothers historically and with all others worldwide experiencing birth at that time (Gaskin, 1977).

Reflection: In your experience, have you noticed pregnant women expressing historical connections as described above?

Connecting with her mother

The connecting relationship with the woman's mother is recognized to have significance in pregnancy and birth (Verny and Kelly, 1982; Rubin, 1984, Price, 1988; Sayers, 1989; Raphael-Lef, 1991; Rich, 1992; Wikman *et al.*, 1992; Rothman, 1994; Magana and Clark, 1995; Hampton, 1995; O'Shea, 1998; Underdown, 1998). Rubin's (1984) research describes the role-model status of the grandmother and the need for women to have contact during pregnancy. This is demonstrated in a recent article discussing the significance of the social support provided by grandmothers, where the author indicates how a woman may want to know more of their childhood history and may subsequently evaluate her mother–daughter relationship (Downe, 1998). Within the western world such a relationship may be distant physically and emotionally, which may make such assessment difficult, and birth itself may reveal hidden negative feelings towards the grandmother (Price, 1988; Sayers, 1989; Raphael-Leff, 1991; Rich, 1992). Eisenstein (1984) goes as far as to suggest that feminists in particular may feel extreme anger at their own mothers for being 'the major agents of their socialization into a passive role'.

This may not apply within other cultural groups, where women are more valued socially and have a supportive role in pregnancy. Complications arise where the woman has two mothers, as in the case of having been adopted (Raphael-Leff, 1991; Hampton, 1995), though it is not known if this may also be applied to women who are born as the result of infertility treatment. Research into birth experiences of twenty adoptees identified a conflict with respect to identification with a mother who gave her child for adoption and with the other mother who was not able to give birth. The researcher suggests that these women had been influenced on a subconscious level by this infertility and that this had affected their self-image when pregnant themselves (Hampton, 1995). When pregnant the inability to develop a connecting relationship with their adoptive mother was due to a poor 'continuity of experience' rather than because of being unable to share. Hampton explains how this is related to the need to hear our mothers' and grandmothers' birth stories. The researcher identified a lack of 'belonging' in these women, which resulted in the majority searching for their natural mother during pregnancy or shortly after birth. It is significant that those who discovered this information prior to birth found the knowledge helpful, and those who did not felt it was a disadvantage. The implication for women generally is that the need to connect with their mothers is significant to the birthing experience, psychologically and spiritually.

Reflection: In your experience, how influential is the woman's relationship with her mother during pregnancy?

Connecting with her partner

In O'Shea's (1998) study some of the women identified connection occurring with their partner through the transformation of the relationship from a couple to a family. These women were all primiparous, and therefore it is not known whether this is only applicable to those couples for whom it is their first child. It is also not known what effect there may be on the spiritual experience if the women do not feel 'connected' to their partners, but alienated, following a child's birth.

Connecting with others

A further aspect of feminine spirituality appears to be the need for women to have connecting relationships with others apart from family (Burkhardt, 1994). The pregnant woman may find her connecting relationships through involvement in antenatal groups, which would indicate that parenting classes may serve another purpose other than providing information. It would be interesting to know if those women who establish a caring, connecting relationship within their parenting class found them more valuable than those who did not. Other sources may be through toddler groups or individual friendships. Often these friendships forged in early pregnancy last a long time.

Reflection: In what ways may antenatal groups be developed to foster connecting and supportive relationships in needy women?

Connecting with the midwife

The physical and emotional effects of female social support in pregnancy, labour and the puerperium have been researched, with the results being mainly positive (Paykel *et al.*, 1980; Sosa *et al.*, 1980; Klaus *et al.*, 1986; Jenner, 1988; Kennell *et al.*, 1991; Oakley, 1992). For the pregnant woman in the UK, the most likely carer she could establish a connecting relationship with is a midwife. In a society where families are apart physically, midwives may take on an increasingly supportive role (Laryea, 1989; Silverton, 1993). Women indicate that they would prefer to have a professional carer with whom they have developed a trusting, caring relationship (Flint and Poulengeris, 1987; Bluff and Holloway, 1994; Halldorsdottir *et al.*, 1996; Page, 1996). Rubin's (1984) research into maternal identity identified that women feel a threat 'to survival and to intactness' when the carer does not know their needs. This would indicate that the need to develop a trusting relationship is more than just a desire for friendship, but is a question of the woman being able to survive living through the experience.

Researchers have identified that women also want a relationship that is not too close, but allows space for the woman to be herself (Halldorsdottir *et al.*, 1996). The writers call this 'professional intimacy', which allows space for the woman being cared for but also allows for 'connection'. In this respect, it would appear that the connecting relationship may be dependent on how the woman is treated by the professional carer, and not just on the structure of maternity services. Flint (1986, p. 1) has suggested that 'a woman never forgets her midwife' and that 'whatever happens to midwives affects women and whatever happens to women affects midwives'. The connecting relationship a woman develops with her midwife may, therefore, affect the midwife as well. A scheme promoting the development of a trusting relationship with one midwife has identified that midwives have greater satisfaction with this method of working, and that it is with the 'meaningful relationship' developed with women that provides this satisfaction (Page, 1996; Sandall, 1997). Sandall concludes her research comparing different schemes of midwifery practice by stating that providing continuity of carer 'is as important to midwives as it is to women'.

The knowledge that midwives and mothers may have differing perceptions of need indicates the difficulties there may be in establishing effective relationships (Laryea, 1989; Goodenough and Barratt, 1991). Goodenough and Barratt (1991) suggest this discrepancy could be reduced through the woman having more time with her midwife for discussion, which would further indicate a need for a relationship to be developed. The inability of the woman to develop a connecting relationship with a known midwife may leave her with a sense of disappointment and discouragement (Berg *et al.*, 1996; Halldorsdottir *et al.*, 1996). Also there is suggestion that the excessive use of technology leads to a sense of separation instead of connection (Davis-Floyd and Davis, 1997).

It is not known whether this ability to develop meaningful relationships is gender specific and related to the femininity of the majority of midwives. Connecting relationships with male midwives may be more difficult, because of the intensity and level of intimacy. However, Rubin's (1984) research based in America, where doctors are the main carers, shows the women building continual relationships with their doctor, though it is not indicated how intense such relationships become.

Reflection: Have you been aware of women developing connect-ing relationships with a carer? In what ways have such relationships been positive or negative?

Connecting with the unborn child

A further connecting relationship that could occur is with the woman's unborn child. Rubin (1984) argues that the child cannot be independent from the way the mother is or how she behaves. Though postnatal attachment between mother and child has been actively researched, it is suggested that a connecting relationship may take place at any time during the pregnancy (Reading and Cox, 1982; Verny and Kelly, 1982; Hebblethwaite, 1984; Schwartz, 1991; LaChance, 1991). Women with high risk or uncertain pregnancies may actively close themselves to becoming emotionally attached to their unborn child until any threat to the pregnancy has passed (McGeary, 1994). Recent research into motherhood over the age of 35 showed that older mothers also experienced less attachment to their unborn child than younger mothers in the middle stages of pregnancy, which the researchers suggest may be related to antenatal screening in the older group (Berryman and Windridge, 1995). It is suggested that the common use of ultrasound in the antenatal period to visualize the fetus has increased the level of physical and emotional attachment that takes place for the mother (Reading and Cox, 1982; Raphael-Leff, 1991; Rothman, 1994) and for the father (Murphy and Hunt, 1997). Rothman (1994) argues that this is detrimental to the mother, as the technology has turned the fetus into a patient, reducing the mother to the 'maternal environment' and preventing attachment until after the ultrasound has shown the fetus to be 'normal'. This indicates that, rather than increasing the attachment of the mother, the use of ultrasound may cause her to question the validity of the feelings of attachment she has already experienced prior to the investigation taking place. However, spiritual connection may take place with or without the use of ultrasound.

Bergum's (1989) phenomenological investigation of the process of women's transformation to motherhood describes the relationship as '. . . peculiar to women who carry within their own bodies the body of another . . .' (p. 53), indicating the 'mysterious union' where the woman and the fetus are one, yet two separate beings. This unity but separateness is identified by Salter (1987), who bases her work on the 'spiritual scientist' Rudolph Steiner. She suggests that, though the parents provide the physical body for the child, the child's spirit 'already is', and early in pregnancy enters the mother, who may then have a dream related to a white bird or light. Others may experience an awareness of the 'presence' of the child around them, a phenomenon also described by Stockley (1986).

Recognizing that the child has a separate identity, or spirit, apart from the mother indicates there is a potential for the child to initiate a connecting relationship which, it has been suggested, may be in the form of dreams (Verny and Kelly, 1982). This may only be enabled if the mother is spiritually receptive and in a spiritually aware environment (Kahn, 1995). Non-receptivity and ambivalence towards the pregnancy by the mother have been documented as possible causes for psychological difficulties in adulthood (Verny and Kelly, 1982; MacNutt and MacNutt, 1988) and miscarriage (Stockley, 1986). This would indicate a need for greater recognition of the connecting relationship between child and mother in utero and how this may be enhanced.

Reflection: In what ways may such a connecting relationship be encouraged? Is it possible to encourage it if it is being facilitated by the child?

Supportive presence

Nursing care involves the physical presence and support of the nurse. For instance, one author (Labun, 1988) writes of caring as being:

- Assertive actions.
- Quiet support.
- Helping to grow.
- Aware of cultural needs.
- Aware of physical preferences.
- Aware of social needs.
- An attitude of helping, sharing, nurturing and loving.

Others have differentiated between the physical 'being there' and the psychological 'being with' (Harrison and Burnard, 1993). However, Osterman and Schwartz-Barcott (1996) have elicited four different descriptions of 'presence' from the nursing literature. These are as follows.

- *Presence*: This is where the nurse is physically in the room with another, but totally self-absorbed, and therefore not available to the other.
- *Partial presence*: This is where the nurse is physically present but focusses her energy on a task rather than the other person.
- *Full presence*: This is where the nurse is physically and psychologically present and each patient interaction is 'personalized'.
- *Transcendent presence*: This is described as 'spiritual' presence and is said to come from a 'spiritual source initiated by centring'. The presence is felt as peaceful, comforting and harmonious. There are seen to be no limits on the role of the nurse and she is able to recognize 'oneness' with the patient.

Comfort and security are also elements given to the client through the real presence of the carer (Bottorff, 1991). Bottorff describes the carer as being able to feel, to share and to understand alongside the client, and thus give them hope. Presence is also described in the context of the person providing spiritual healing (Brown, 1998).

Burkhardt (1998) further describes the conscious act of letting go of the concerns of the person she has left in order to be fully aware and present for the person that she next encounters. She states that being 'truly present' means:

- Seeing and hearing with eyes, ears and heart.
- Trusting intuition.
- Using cognitive evaluation.

   Reflection: Do you recognize a difference between 'being there' with someone and truly 'being with' them?

The midwife with presence

For midwives the meanings of presence carry significance, as the Anglo-Saxon meaning of the title 'midwife' is 'with woman' (Flint, 1986). Research has shown that the supportive presence of a midwife is beneficial to women, and may lead to enhancement of their role as mothers (Flint and Poulengeris, 1987; Evans, 1991; Oakley, 1992). Further, the concept of continuity of carer allows the development of a relationship which is beneficial to both the woman and her midwife (Page, 1996; Sandall, 1997). Halldorsdottir *et al.*'s (1996) research of women's experience of caring by midwives demonstrated that effective support is given through:

- Competent ability.
- True concern for a woman.
- A favourable mental attitude.

The positive relationship described between a woman and her midwife is one of intimate professionalism but where respect and compassion enable a safe distance. Berg *et al.* (1996), also studying women's experiences of their midwife, illustrated the phenomenon of 'presence' and argue that it is necessary to enable a favourable interaction to occur. They suggest that this presence pervades the encounter with the following needs:

- To be seen as an individual.
- To have a dependable relationship.
- To have support and be directed on one's own conditions.

Negatively, they suggest that some midwives were unable to provide this relationship, and were described as 'absently present'.

From this information it could be surmised that midwives are in a position to provide the supportive presence required in effective spiritual care, but that this support needs to be more than just the provision of physical presence and care. For the women in O'Shea's (1998) study, the midwives concerned were described as being 'emotionally involved' in their care. In describing the therapeutic value of the midwife/woman relationship, Siddiqui (1999) elicits that there should be:

- Authenticity of being
- Conscience
- Commitment
- Presence
- Compassion
- Empathy
- Empowerment.

From this it is apparent that the relationship aspect of midwifery care is significant, and can enhance the woman's self-esteem, as well as encouraging the midwife to give the type of support the women require (Flint and Poulengeris, 1987; Oakley, 1992; Sandall, 1997).

Case history 4

Carrie had been admitted to the labour ward of the hospital having been in the first stage of labour for over 24 hours at home. She had desperately wanted a home birth for this, her second child, but she seemed to have got 'stuck' with the cervix at 7 cm dilated and couldn't go any further. Her community midwife had tried everything to help her, but there seemed to be nothing more that she could do. The community midwife had come in with her but felt she should hand over Carrie's care to another midwife – a 'fresh face' to help support her through the next stage. Carrie and her partner were feeling very tired and fed up. She had required augmentation with syntocinon with her last labour and had ended up with an epidural and a forceps delivery. She had desperately wanted everything normal. She was also disappointed that the community midwife was going and concerned that the hospital midwife would make her do things she didn't want. When the community midwife had handed over care, Sarah, the labour ward midwife, went in to see Carrie. She was lying on the bed looking very miserable. The contractions had slowed down to 5 minutes apart and were not very strong. Sarah introduced herself and then discussed some options with Carrie. She suggested having a rest, having some breakfast, relaxing in the birthing pool, getting the contractions going again with stimulation of her nipples, or a combination of all of them. Carrie was very surprised -- she had thought the midwife would have put up a drip straight away! She brightened up immediately as the midwife encouraged her by saying that she was sure Carrie could give birth on her own and that she wanted to help her. The warmth and response that Carrie felt resulted in the contractions starting again. She decided that resting was not what she wanted to do and Sarah helped her to stand upright and lean against the bed. For the next hour Sarah concentrated on supporting Carrie through the contractions, looking frequently into her eyes to tell her that she could do it, until the baby at last was visible. Carrie gave birth to a healthy girl while she was standing up. Afterwards, she told Sarah that she had been very fearful of getting 'stuck' in labour this time. She said that the community midwife had been nice, but that she always felt she was busy and had her mind on other things, even when Carrie was in labour. When she had reached 6 cm this time, the midwife had been persuading her to go to hospital by saying 'I don't think you'll push this baby out – it's bigger than the last'. Carrie said it had made her feel like giving up. Carrie said, in contrast, that when Sarah had given her choices and told her she could give birth, she had felt supported and felt that Sarah had been totally concentrating on her and was 'with' her in the experience. She said she wished Sarah had been at home with her! Carrie was able to go home with her new baby within a few hours of giving birth.

Reflection: Is it feasible to expect every midwife to have the type of relationship described above with every woman in their care?

Conclusion

During pregnancy a woman may desire or aim to belong and she may manifest this through involvement in religious, social or political groups. A woman may also establish 'connecting' relationships with:

- Women of history
- Her mother
- Her partner
- The midwife
- The unborn child.

A woman may attach great significance and meaning to these relationships, and an integral part of midwifery care may be to encourage and support the woman as she moves through this process. For this a midwife will need to develop a relationship that will enable her to be truly 'present' with the woman. Whether it is feasible to expect this kind of relationship with every woman a midwife cares for is a matter for speculation. However, there may be particular situations where such 'connection' may take place so as to enable effective 'presence' as well.

Relationship and the compassionate midwife

Relational aspects

As addressed in the previous chapter, definitions of spirituality have also included aspects of relationship other than belonging and connecting, such as being able to give and receive love and practical care giving. These issues are relevant to women because of the potential of a loving and giving relationship with partners and children.

Pregnancy

Rubin's (1984) research into maternal experience recognizes this giving relationship. She states that the process of becoming pregnant is an act of the woman giving of herself for another: firstly, to give a child to her partner and then to family and to society. She suggests that by doing this the woman lets go of her 'physical, mental and social self'. But it also involves the process of giving life to another, through the pregnancy and through the act of birth itself.

Sered's (1991) study of women of Jewish faith showed that many women felt that their spiritual experience was in the development of their relationship with their baby, rather than in the physical experiences. The giving of themselves to the relationship leads to accepting a 'responsibility of caring' which may result in changing behaviour patterns to protect or enhance that care (Sered, 1991; McGeary, 1994). This change in behaviour linked to a new life within highlights the sacrificial nature of the mother, and is often used as a key by health professionals to encourage a modification of unsociable behaviour (e.g. smoking or drinking alcohol). The mother is expected to give all for the sake of the child.

Birth

The phrase 'giving birth' is used to describe the point at which the child enters the world. Whereas in medical involvement birth is described in terms of 'delivery', in the normal process language identifies the mother as needing to be part of the action, as needing to give life to her child. Bergum's (1989) study into women's transformation to motherhood suggests that labour and birth are an opportunity for a woman's growth and that she should have an opportunity for deliberation on what she has gone through with those who had been present with her at the birth.

Women's recognition of their need to participate fully in the birth of their child has led to an increased desire to experience a natural labour (Gaskin, 1977; Hebblethwaite, 1984; Kahn, 1995; Belbin, 1996). Disappointment, and more severely a form of post-traumatic stress, may then be experienced if this is not achieved (Knight *et al.*, 1987 cited in Sherr, 1995; Price, 1988; Rich, 1992; Allott, 1996; Menage, 1996). In describing the spiritual aspects of birth, Stockley (1986) suggests that, with good preparation, it is possible to have a spiritual experience with any birth, but also implies that having spiritual awareness may lead to a more natural labour. She also indicates that some medical interventions may interfere with the spiritual process and subsequently affect the physical aspects. Interventions into the expected natural process have led some women to describe feelings of failure in themselves as women, and others have feelings of anger at the failure of the system to support them (Rich, 1992; Halldorsdottir *et al.*, 1994). If the experience was also expected to be spiritual, then this could be regarded as a failure in the spiritual quest, leading to development of spiritual distress (Smucker, 1996). The expectation of natural childbirth could therefore lead to either positive or negative experiences. Bergum (1989) insinuates that the action of the woman giving birth in a positive way physically, emotionally and spiritually will have long-term implications for the future of society.

Reflection: In your opinion do those women who opt for a more natural birth act in a more spiritual way or are they made to because of the normality of the experience?

Love

There is an expectation that the mother and child will have a relationship based on love. The social expectation is that this love will occur immediately. For some women this may develop during pregnancy while for others the process of 'falling in love' with the child will happen much later. For some women the desire to bear a child is to meet a need of love, to have someone who will give them love in return (Gittens, 1985; Price, 1988; Raphael-Leff, 1991). Pregnancy develops usually as a result of love between two people, and involves the woman in the giving of herself to pregnancy as a result of her love for her partner (Rubin, 1984). Love is identified as a powerful spiritual force linked with pregnancy, the birth of the child, and subsequently the act of breastfeeding.

Love during pregnancy

In pregnancy the love of the mother for the child may show through her changing her lifestyle to meet the needs of the child (Rubin, 1984; Bergum, 1989; Raphael-Leff, 1991). Research has suggested that the unborn child both sees and hears in the womb (Verny and Kelly, 1982; Schwartz, 1991), and that he may recognize emotionally when he is unwanted or rejected by the mother (Verny and Kelly, 1982). If this is true, then conversely, he may also recognize when he is loved and wanted. Salter (1987) suggests that, in societies where instinctive mothering has been lost, pregnant women should spend 10 to 15 minutes each day reflecting on their unborn child. Others have suggested that the parents pray for, talk to and sing to their unborn child as a sign of their love (MacNutt and MacNutt, 1988).

Love after birth

Following birth a loving response in the mother may be triggered by the sight of the large size of the baby's eyes and its vulnerability, and the sound of the baby's cry (Gaskin, 1987; Morris, 1991; Odent, 1994). It is further suggested that the sight of the baby's smile is a responding signal of love (Rubin, 1984). As a new mother, Bloom (1981, p. 260) describes her feelings of love as 'a powerful, natural, hormonal, physical, sexual, mystical "high"', in which she possesses 'heightened consciousness and increased powers of observation and impressionability'. The responses of love may have a physical basis, in that a surge of the release of oxytocin in the mother just after the birth of the baby may have an effect on the loving response of the mother. This, combined with the presence of endorphins, may give a sense of dependency (Odent, 1994). The physical response of a woman is for her to look at the child, usually naked, and then stroke and caress it (Rubin, 1984; Gaskin, 1987; Morris, 1991; Raphael-Leff, 1991; Fraser, 1997). Flint (1986) suggests encouraging such behaviour to enhance love in mothers who are having difficulty in establishing a relationship. The participants in O'Shea's (1998) study all described the love and closeness they felt towards their babies. Some felt they could 'die for their baby', but that it was also something that grew over time rather than a 'rush of emotion'. A woman describing her full-term stillbirth spoke of an experience of love unlike any other she had felt before. This shows that the love experienced was real and intense despite there being no physical or emotional response from the child.

Reflection: In your opinion is a loving relationship with a baby just physical and emotional or is it always spiritual?

Breastfeeding as an act of love

The intensity of the relationship that develops through the intimacy of breastfeeding may be an indication of the love that has developed pre- and postnatally (Verny and Kelly, 1982; Gittens, 1985). In Rubin's (1984) study into maternal experience, feeding is described as an important aspect of the interactive development between mother and infant. She uses the words 'working intensely', 'concentrated effort' and 'earnestness' to describe the new mother's aims 'to achieve goodness of fit' in meeting the needs of her child. These efforts may be as a result of the depth of love the mother feels. A study described by Verny and Kelly (1982) indicates that mothers who form a deep bond with their child may have a more enjoyable experience of breastfeeding and will breastfeed longer than those mothers who do not form such a bond. It has also been shown that there is a link between women's satisfaction with motherhood 6 weeks after the birth and breastfeeding their baby within an hour of birth (Ball, 1994). The experience of breastfeeding has also been described in the context of 'romantic' love, and the intensity and intimacy of a relationship that must ultimately end through weaning (Bloom, 1981). Bloom relates feeding to the concept of power and the mother's ability to create, nurture and empower a child. She suggests that this ability '. . . reaffirms, through the love of her child, her sexual power as a woman and her political and professional power as a person'. She indicates that the ability of a mother to feed is powerful, and that the power comes from love.

This element of power may also be a cause of conflict in the love relationship between the woman and her partner. The exclusivity of the act of breastfeeding, and the intensity of the maternal love, may be a source of a father's jealousy of the child (Gittens, 1985). The hormonal balance in the mother may also have an influence on this situation. Odent (1995) argues that the low levels of prolactin present when not breastfeeding will focus a woman's love towards her sexual partner, whereas if there are high levels because she is breastfeeding she will direct her love more to her baby due to the depressing effect of the hormone on sexual arousal.

Reflection: Does this information indicate that those who do not choose to breastfeed are less loving mothers or that those who breastfeed long term are too loving?

The feelings associated with love should not be isolated to just a reaction to hormones. The issues raised in the previous chapter relating to belief and acceptance of unconditional love, placing value on others and being able to receive love may increase a woman's ability to give love to her child. Though not proven, such elements of giving worth and support may be real factors in enabling her to feel safe to give to her child.

Reflection: Are there other ways a woman may feel supported in order to be able to give love to her child?

Understanding

Spiritual care requires understanding to be:

- Non-judgemental (Dickinson, 1975).
- Affirming (Price *et al.*, 1995).

• Able to recognize the personal views of the person being cared for (Labun, 1988).

Empathy

Empathy may also be included under this heading and has been defined as: 'the ability to perceive the meanings and feelings of another person and communicate that understanding to the other' (Gagan, 1983, cited in Olsen, 1991, p. 63). It is then suggested that empathy between two people is based on feeling the same because of both being human (Olsen, 1991). Within midwifery this empathy could also arise through sharing the common bond of femininity which may not occur in the case of male midwives, or through the bond of motherhood where the midwife has experienced birth herself. Where the midwife has had a negative experience of birth, her understanding may be limited to that experience, and she may therefore be unable to empathize with others whose experiences differ.

In relating empathy to the therapeutic relationship of the midwife, it is seen to require the midwife to be intuitive, with the woman then being able to show the depth of her understanding of another person (Siddiqui, 1999). It is further argued that the empathetic midwife serves as a role model for others in promoting the 'artistry of midwifery at its highest level'. Empathy is thus seen as being essential for the effective provision of midwifery care.

> *Reflection: Is the ability to be empathetic essential to effective care, as suggested here? Which midwives appear to be most able to be empathetic to the experiences of the women in their care?*

Empathy through touch

It has been suggested that empathy can be expressed through sensitive touch (Dickinson, 1975). In midwifery, as in any form of care, skill is required to be able to judge when touch is appropriate. It is suggested that physical change can take place through the touch of the midwife (Gaskin, 1977) and the caring touch is not only physical in nature, but also has the potential to touch the inner person (Bottorff, 1991). Touch may also be an aspect of spiritual healing (Brown, 1998). However, in contrast, inappropriate or insensitive touch, or touch that is restricted when expected, may have deeply negative effects (Kahn, 1995; Berg *et al.*, 1996; Halldorsdottir *et al.*, 1996; Kitzinger, 1997).

Kitzinger (1997) helpfully provides a classification of different forms of touch during childbirth. These are:

• *The blessing touch*: She describes this as being one where the birth attendant has a recognized spiritual function or power, and will use physical contact accompanied by prayers or other spiritual rites, or methods of massage, to assist the birth process.

- *The comfort touch*: She describes this as being methods of touch, such as massage or caressing, involved to provide support or enable pain relief, but in the context of the continuous presence and support of female companionship.
- *Physically supportive touch*: She describes this as activity involved in encouraging movement or change of position to enable the birth process.
- *Diagnostic touch*: She describes as the skills used to identify and evaluate the state of the pregnancy or birth progress through the use of eyes, ears and hands.
- *Manipulative touch*: She describes this as the use of a midwife's hands to enable healing or manipulation to assist the birth process.
- *Restraining touch*: A negative form which she describes as methods used to keep a woman immobile, or unable to interfere with examinations or medical processes.
- *Punitive touch*: A more negative form which she describes as violent methods used to 'punish' a woman who attempts to interfere with medical control. She also describes this in the context of situations where women perceive investigations, such as vaginal examinations, as being violent acts.

These demonstrate that a midwife's methods of touch in labour are vitally important for the woman concerned and care needs to be taken as to how this is perceived. Kitzinger (1997) concludes that touch will either be 'emotionally supportive or disabling', which suggests that a midwife through her touch has much responsibility for the spiritual experience of the woman.

Reflection: Compare the types of touch described above with how you use touch or how you see others use touch. Can you identify where touch has had a positive or negative effect?

Understanding through relationships

True understanding may only be developed over a period of time through establishing a relationship. In midwifery relationships between woman and midwife have developed most effectively in schemes where woman-centred care has been established (Flint and Poulengeris, 1987; Evans, 1991; Page, 1996; Sandall, 1997). In recent studies the women investigated recognized understanding as a midwife's skill, and also recognized when they did not feel this understanding to be present (Berg *et al.*, 1996; Halldorsdottir *et al.*, 1996). The lack of understanding was perceived to be uncaring and not beneficial to the woman. From this it could be supposed that understanding which is communicated and received mutually, i.e. empathetic understanding (Olsen 1991), is that which is required to administer effective spiritual care in midwifery.

The midwife with love and compassion

In the English language there is one word to describe many aspects of 'love', while other languages have different words giving different meaning (Rawlings, 1995). Consequently, the concept of 'love' could mean different things to different people. Within spiritual care, loving is recognized as a nursing action (Dickinson, 1975; Gaskin, 1977; Fish and Shelly, 1978; Labun, 1988; Allen, 1991), and spiritual healers channel love from a higher source to their patient (Brown, 1998). Bottorff (1991) also equates caring with giving love but includes that the carer must also be prepared to 'suffer with others'. Thus, the depth of care this signifies is expressed by recognizing the worth of the individual and wanting to give the best for her, without expecting anything in return. Clarke (1996) describes this as the concept of 'unconditional love', and suggests for midwives that this is an essential part of care. She recommends that midwives evaluate their relationships with women and assess if they accept and recognize the worth of the women in their care. Flint (1986) also signifies recognizing value through her use of the word 'cherish' in respect of both the midwife loving herself and in loving her client. Giving 'genuine concern and respect', which could be recognized as a loving action, is also a trait of the caring midwife (Halldorsdottir et al., 1996).

> Reflection: In what ways do midwives demonstrate 'love' of their clients? What effect does this love have?

Gaskin's (1977) concept of the spiritual midwife requires her to love women deeply and each person equally. She highlights 'compassion and spiritual vision' as essential components of this loving. Rawlings (1995) also expresses care in the terms of love and compassion, and suggests that their use enables a 'stronger foundation on which the lives of future generations can be built'. This implies that the act of the midwife giving love to a woman enables a strengthening of love within the woman toward her child. Therefore, if a spiritual self-development takes place in a woman during the transformation to motherhood, as explored previously, then the loving care of a midwife may facilitate or be a part of this process.

> Reflection: In what ways may compassion be developed? Does a midwife loving a woman encourage loving of the child?

> Reflection: Can you recognize times where love in action has been demonstrated and been effective?

Conclusion

The issues of love and relationship are significant for the pregnant woman and new mother and for those caring for her. From a spiritual perspective the ability to give and receive love may be regarded as positive signs of the presence of spiritual well-being. To this end a midwife's role will be to encourage this ability in a woman as well as giving and caring for her in a loving way. This love may be demonstrated through:

- Empathy and understanding.
- Attentive listening and meeting needs.
- Appropriate, gentle, physical touch.
- Development of a relationship with the woman.

This sort of love may be enabled through provision of continuity in those who care for a woman (Flint and Poulengeris, 1987). The attitude of the midwife carries significance (Clarke, 1996), and she also may find it easier to love if she feels loved, valued and cared for herself (Flint, 1986).

To enable a woman to love her child she may be encouraged and supported in:

- Focussing on her unborn child during pregnancy, such as through prayer, talking or singing to him.
- Spending time with the newborn infant with skin-to-skin contact, stroking and caressing, and having time just to look at him.
- Breastfeeding as an act of love.

7 *Development of self and the self-aware midwife*

Self-development

As highlighted in Chapter 2 the concepts of 'self' and self-development have been identified by others as elements of spirituality. In the context of pregnancy and the transformation to motherhood, changes take place in the woman physically and emotionally, with accompanying sociological change. It is appropriate to suggest that spiritual change to the 'self' will also evolve. Belenky *et al.*'s (1986) study of women's self-development showed that many women identified childbirth as the most important learning experience in their lives. They linked the creative act with a greater understanding of the woman's ability to be creative. The creative nature of the experience, and the participation of the woman in it, has also been identified by others as relevant to women's experiences (Bergum, 1989; Sokoloski, 1995; Khalaf and Callister, 1997; O'Shea, 1998).

Transformation through giving birth

Through her study into maternal identity, Rubin (1984) establishes that there is a transformation that evolves in the maternal self over time in pregnancy and into the puerperium. She suggests that 'childbearing requires an exchange of a known self in a known world for an unknown self in an unknown world' (p. 52). This 'exchange' and self-growth may be particularly apparent during the act of birth itself, which has been related to the achievement of climbing a mountain and the woman being able to recognize in herself a greater strength and ability (Bergum, 1989). Within this act pain is identified as a positive element for achieving self-knowledge. Bergum states: 'As women give birth to children, they, in a sense, birth themselves' (p. 81). This latter statement was also used by Rich (1992) in describing her own experiences of changing into being a mother. During childbirth it is suggested (Hampton, 1995) that a woman will have to face her:

- Self
- Fears
- Joys
- Connections
- Separations.

It has also been suggested that women encounter their 'wild' selves through the experiences of pregnancy, breastfeeding and the changes of motherhood (Estes, 1992).

From these statements it could be surmised that with the self-development that evolves birth may be always a spiritual event. However, the women investigated for Sered's (1991) study tended to experience the spiritual aspects after the actual birth, viewing the birth more from the physical aspect alone. It has been argued that for 'creative growth' to take place, women need to have developed some self-awareness prior to pregnancy (Price, 1988). In O'Shea's (1998) pilot study the multiparous women interviewed preferred to talk more of their first birth, as it was the one best remembered because it involved the most emotional experience. However, it may be that one birth is more spiritual than another, or that the woman is more receptive to spirituality during one birth than another. For instance, Rich (1992) writes of the birth of her first child as being a 'psychic crisis', while LaChance (1991) identifies her second birth as transforming: 'Whereas my first experience of birth was a rite of passage into motherhood, this birth was a rite of passage into my self as mother' (p. 12).

Bergum (1989), in her study of the transformation of motherhood, questions if women become themselves through becoming a mother. In contrast, King (1993) suggests such an idea to be too 'body-dependent' and traditional, and identifies that single, childless women are able to make great contributions to society through their own experiences. It is also suggested that some women experience a form of grief at the loss of her previous self before motherhood (Speck, 1988). Though it may not be necessary for a woman to become a mother to achieve self-awareness, it is apparent that there is a change, or self-growth, that occurs in women who become mothers that is probably spiritual, as well as physical and psychological. The 'self' as woman becomes 'self with child', firstly through the adjustment of pregnancy, and then once the child is born. It has been suggested that: 'The separation that occurs in childbirth makes possible the wholeness of both mother and child' (Bergum, 1989, p. 155). How this relates to those who give birth but do not have a live child is arguable. Is it the act of birth that gives the 'wholeness' or the having of the child?

The connecting relationship with the child is very complex, and the relationships of the self in context with her partner, family and the social community are adjusted as a consequence (Rubin, 1984). It is suggested that: 'A mother who lacks a sense of self will tend to merge with her child in a way that prevents both from developing' (Dally, 1982, p. 199). This growth of self appears to be enhanced if the mother is in contact with empathetic, caring, affirming and supportive midwives (Gaskin, 1977; Flint, 1986, 1987; Goodenough and Barratt, 1991; Ball, 1994; Belbin, 1996; Berg et al., 1996; Halldorsdottir and Karlsdottir, 1996). Waugh's (1992) study of nurses' spiritual perceptions identified that spiritual care was dependent on the spiritual awareness and sensitivity of particular nurses. The lack of research into midwives' care makes a comparison difficult. However, Goodenough and Barratt's (1991) study into perceptions of the transition into motherhood identified that midwives who were able to have a 'self' perspective were able to identify more closely with the women in their care. This would suggest that a midwife should have an element of self-growth in order to facilitate growth of self-awareness in a woman.

Reflection: Have you been aware of 'growth' in women during pregnancy or labour that you would regard as 'transformation'? Is this more pronounced in first pregnancies/births? What factors have facilitated such growth?

Case history 4

To illustrate this issue of self-growth, the reader is recommended the story of Alison Belbin and the birth of her son Eddie (Belbin, 1996). From her perspective, the experience of giving birth enhanced her 'self-esteem' and gave her strength and confidence in her mothering skills. She also highlighted the support of a particular midwife as crucial to the positive outcomes of the experience. This midwife, through her support of Alison's wishes and positive language, enabled Alison to grow in her self-confidence and belief in herself. The study demonstrates how positive midwifery care can provide women with the elements required for self-growth.

The midwife with spiritual self-awareness

It has been suggested that it is not possible for a carer to give spiritual care unless she has an awareness of her own spirituality, with or without religious belief, and has her own spiritual needs met (Myco, 1985; Carson, 1989a; McSherry, 1996; O'Shea, 1998). It has been argued that nurses should recognize the 'values and beliefs' they hold (Harrison and Burnard, 1993) and that they should also know their own limitations in understanding others' beliefs (Labun, 1988). A study relating to the spiritual care given by a group of nurses with Christian beliefs demonstrated that comfort with giving spiritual care was dependent on the age of the nurse and length of time they had held their beliefs (Hall and Lanig, 1993). From this the authors argue that nurses should not be expected to give spiritual care until they are prepared themselves. Waugh (1992) also identified in her study of nurses' perceptions of spiritual care that those who had more awareness of spiritual care had an awareness of their own spirituality.

The results of giving care

A study of perceptions of what nursing care means showed that the nurses gave of themselves but also received something back through doing so (Clarke and Wheeler, 1992). It is suggested elsewhere that those who give spiritual care may also benefit from it through release of tension, and that spiritual growth will subconsciously take place (Kaye and Robinson, 1994; Price *et al.*, 1995). It is also surmised that such care could result in a reduction in nurse 'burn-out' (Price *et al.*, 1995). Others have intimated that by providing spiritual care to others, the carer will be 'replenished' spiritually themselves (Brown-Salzman, 1997). Being spiritually aware may therefore bring positive experiences to both client and carer.

For midwives, Gaskin (1977) argues that the 'holiness' of the event of birth requires the midwife to be spiritually aware and living a religious life. She states that a midwife should be constantly examining her habits and be prepared to change her life to remain spiritually 'in top condition'. This intensity may be offensive to those without religious belief; however, there remains a need to recognize the spiritual potential within the birth process, and to meet the needs of pregnant and birthing women. O'Shea (1998) argues for midwives who will not be 'threatened' by the spiritual needs of these women.

It is further suggested that midwives will be unable to care effectively for women unless they receive love, 'cherishing' and care themselves (Flint, 1986). The need for love is identified as a spiritual need (Fish and Shelly, 1978; Highfield and Cason, 1983). This would indicate that to be spiritually effective midwives should have their own spiritual needs met. If, as suggested, spiritual forms of care result in less symptoms of carer 'burn-out', the results of Sandall's (1997) study into midwives' stress, as related to schemes providing continuity of care, indicate that what is also required is a midwife who is:

- Able to ascertain her personal needs and be assertive about meeting them.
- Secure and supported in her home and workplace relationships.
- Able to form meaningful relationships with the women in her care.

This suggests self-awareness, and though primarily based on physical and emotional information, this may also be applicable in the spiritual sense.

Reflection: Does a midwife have to be spiritually aware in order to be able to provide spiritual care to others? How may this be encouraged in colleagues?

Conclusion

This chapter has focussed on self-development as an element of spirituality. Though some would suggest that this is a remit of psychology and its influence, it could be argued that, if we are spiritual people, then spirituality must also be an aspect of the self. With this in mind, pregnancy and birth have been noted as a time of transformation for women and could be regarded as a potential time of spiritual growth. The act of giving birth itself is particularly significant, due to the powerful process of creativity that takes place. Women are enabled in this process of growth by the presence of caring, supportive midwives with characteristics of empathy. Midwives have also been suggested to require awareness of their own spirituality and the need to give spiritual care before they are able to be truly effective.

⑧ Intuition and the intuitive midwife

Intuition and the mother

In the provision of spiritual care the skill of intuition has been argued to be a major element (Gaskin, 1977; Waugh, 1992; Harrison and Burnard, 1993). As we are discussing the context of woman as carer to her child it is relevant to approach intuition as a possible component of her spirituality. As outlined in Chapter 2, intuitive 'knowing' has been argued to be a particular element of spirituality related to women. In high technology, developed societies this form of knowledge has less value placed on it because of the inability to demonstrate it in a scientific way, while in more traditional societies it may be more accepted (Belenky *et al.*, 1986). Within these societies instinctive mothering may be more commonplace because of the ability of women to trust their senses (Verny and Kelly, 1982; Salter, 1987). However, it has been suggested that intuition is a skill that can be learned and that pregnant women may be particularly intuitive if 'allowed' to be (Stockley, 1986). During labour, Stockley states that a woman can be helped to be intuitive by:

- Loving and constant support (preferably from someone known).
- Listening carefully to her for her wants and needs.
- Reducing or removing 'outside interference, noise or obstruction'.

The provision of support from a known carer is identified as having a significantly positive effect upon the woman's well-being. Holistically, it could be supposed that this will also include the spiritual aspect, as Stockley suggests.

> *Reflection: Have you identified evidence of intuitive behaviours in women during labour?*

Women may experience intuitive behaviour through 'knowing' there is something 'not right' with their child, either before or after birth. Breastfeeding women describe experiences of waking just prior to the child waking for a feed, though hormonal influences may also play a part in this phenomenon. It is identified too, that some African women exhibit intuitive behaviour by 'knowing' when their babies, who are without nappies, need to urinate or defaecate (Pearce, 1972 cited in Stockley, 1986; Verny and Kelly, 1982). The reasons for the latter may also be physical, since the babies are carried on the women's backs or fronts, and the signs may be learned through experience.

Case history 6

As a midwife working on night duty I frequently observed the phenomenon of breastfeeding women in shared rooms waking seconds before their own baby woke for a feed. They were often not disturbed by other babies' cries, but only seemed to respond to their own. Later I experienced this myself with each of my children. I would awaken from a deep sleep into silence, only to hear the baby stirring within seconds. Is this a purely physical response, a hormonal response or intuition? If it is the former, how does the mechanism work? This is something that is very difficult to research or completely explain. Even more difficult to explain are the times when I have been apart from my children and have felt my breast fill – the 'let-down' reflex. On noting the time this happened and discussing it with the child's carer later, invariably this response occurred at the time my child required feeding. Again, is this a completely physical response from a distance, without seeing or hearing the baby cry, or an in-built mechanism of instinct: my spirit and body responding to my daughter's needs?

Reflection: Have you been aware of women behaving intuitively in the caring of their babies? How may this be supported and encouraged?

Intuitive care and openness

Some issues surrounding the subject of intuition have been discussed in respect of a woman's caring relationship with her child. It is also necessary to discuss it in relation to the midwife, as intuitive care has been identified as an element of spiritual care (see Table 1.2). Rew (1989) suggests that this concept is 'central to holistic nursing practice', and situations have been described where nurses and midwives have acted intuitively (Harrison and Burnard, 1993; Davis-Floyd and Davis, 1997). It has been suggested that instinctive nursing care develops through the carer having the confidence and knowledge of being cared for themselves (Clarke and Wheeler, 1992). This would imply the need for personal development to have taken place within the carer, leading to a sense of security within self and relationships.

Connected with intuition is a need for spiritual openness, in order to be able to be guided by a 'sixth sense' (Harrison and Burnard, 1993), or to listen to 'that still small voice' (Allen, 1991). Stockley (1986) states that intuition is a skill that can be learned, and it is suggested that educators could be involved in teaching the skill to nurses (Price *et al.*, 1995). Rew (1989) recommends specific exercises to practise intuition.

Reflection: Is there a place for intuitive practice?

Intuitive midwifery practice

Within midwifery intuition is recognized as a skill, with the spiritual midwife using '. . . the millenia-old, God-given insights and intuition as her tools – in addition to, but often in place of, the hospital's technology, drugs and equipment' (Gaskin, 1977, p. 283). It is suggested that midwives may already use intuitive skills but be unable to put into words how they do so (Siddiqui, 1999). Within our present highly technological midwifery practice this inability may be related to fear of being derided by others.

Reflection: Have you experienced intuition in practice? Have you been able to communicate the experience to your colleagues?

Case history 7

Anna is a midwife working on a mixed antenatal and postnatal ward. One of the women she is caring for, Eleanor, has been admitted for induction of labour, as her pregnancy has stretched on for 14 days over the estimated due date. Anna has been responsible for Eleanor's care, and she administered a dose of Prostin gel to induce the labour about 4 hours ago. The immediate cardiotochograph trace of the fetal heart had been reactive, with few signs of uterine activity. During the hours since then, Eleanor has been wandering around the ward and has had some lunch. Anna has regularly listened to the fetal heartbeat, and all has appeared well, without signs of labour.

Anna goes to Eleanor again and discovers she is now experiencing mild contractions every 15 minutes. She listens again to the heartbeat and it still sounds strong and regular. She recommends that Eleanor gets up and continues to wait for events to happen. She walks out of the room, then suddenly stops and goes back in. She asks Eleanor if she can listen to the fetal heart again. Surprised, Eleanor lies back and Anna picks up the stethoscope. Initially, the heartbeat is strong, but then Anna realizes it is slowing and becoming more faint. She summons help and within minutes Eleanor is in the operating theatre undergoing an emergency caesarean section. At birth the baby does not breathe spontaneously but responds to ventilation. It is discovered that a placental abruption has occurred. Anna's instinct to return and check the heart again had saved the baby's life.

In this dramatic story, Anna was willing and able to follow her intuition enough to act on what could have been regarded as an illogical or irrational 'feeling'. We are left wondering what would have happened if she had not obeyed that 'inner voice' to go back. Further illustrations of this skill are described by Robbie Davis-Floyd and Elizabeth Davis (1997), where they relate interviews with some American midwives talking about their intuitive experiences.

In a less dramatic way, I have experienced this phenomenon myself with the friend who was my midwife for my first labour. I can remember that few contractions were happening and I was not 'in labour' as such but wanted to telephone to warn her that I thought something was going on. I went to pick up the phone, but she was there on the doorstep! It was right that she was, too, in that I gave birth within 3 hours! For my third birth, where we had moved away, she telephoned instinctively as I went into labour. We still have some kind of instinctive bond now, as we often telephone as the other is going to. I believe there is something in my spirit that intuitively connects with something in her in order to behave this way. From a colleague's view, she is one of the most intuitive midwives that I know.

This skill may develop over time, through experience and trusting the ability of women's bodies to be able to give birth, or it may be enhanced through the development of a relationship with a particular woman (Rew, 1989). It is suggested that those midwives specifically involved in home birth and committed to providing holistic care, tend to rely more on intuition than those involved in technological situations. It is also suggested, however, that this skill develops from the ability of the midwife to establish connecting relationships with women and from her own 'internal connectedness' (Davis, 1995; Davis-Floyd and Davis, 1997). What is not known is whether those midwives who are particularly intuitive tend to opt more for that method of care, or whether such intuition develops through practice without relying on technology.

Two recent studies relating to women's experiences of their relationships with midwives both highlighted that women recognize when midwives are practising intuitively (Berg et al., 1996; Halldorsdottir et al., 1996). Berg's study also suggested that such abilities were important to the women, and lack of intuitive care resulted in a loss of the woman's confidence. In these studies a question that could be asked is if the midwives who gave intuitive care were naturally perceptive or particularly spiritually aware. Certainly in Waugh's (1992) study, those who gave more effective spiritual care were identified to have more sensitivity and perception. But they also had an awareness of spiritual matters in themselves and others. What is not known is whether the intuition developed as a result of this awareness, or whether it is an ability that is more apparent in some than in others.

Reflection: Are those midwives you know who appear to practise intuitively more spiritually aware? Are those who are more spiritually aware able to practise intuitively?

The relational aspect of intuition indicates that the phenomenon may only be experienced when caring for particular people and is related to an empathetic bond (Rew, 1989; Davis-Floyd and Davis, 1997). The suggestion that intuition is aided by knowledge developed through a relationship would indicate another beneficial element of providing a known midwife to care for a woman through pregnancy. At the present time, the use of intuitive skills is generally in opposition to the highly technological, evidence-based culture that has developed in midwifery care. It will take time to redress the balance and train midwives who will be able to be reliant on their own hands, eyes, ears and instincts before turning to technology for confirmation.

Reflection: In your experience is it easier to practise intuitively with women you have got to know? How may intuition be taught to others?

Conclusion

This chapter has addressed intuition in relation to the woman in labour and as carer for her child, and in relation to the midwife in how she cares for pregnant women. For the woman the ability to have intuition may enable her:

- To have a deeper sense of her own body, especially during labour.
- To develop a strong relationship with her child.
- To have greater confidence in herself, as she is able to trust her own instincts more.

A midwife who practises in an intuitive way may enhance the care by:

- Developing connecting relationships.
- Developing organizational schemes of care which encourage continuity of the caring relationship.

- Being prepared to use midwifery observational skills before technology, with the aim of enhancing these skills.
- Being prepared to listen to inner instincts and then acting on them.

If this is to be encouraged, midwives in practice need to be more open and willing to discuss how they make decisions about care without fear of being derided by colleagues. Within education the subject also needs to be approached with the aim of developing intuitive skills in students. Until the dialogue begins, intuition will continue to be undervalued or thought of as irrelevant within the current climate of midwifery.

⑨ *Telling stories and the midwife who listens*

Story-telling: the woman's story

In Chapter 2 it was indicated that story-telling may be part of women's spirituality. Following from this it may be suggested to be an aspect of childbirth and women's experiences as a whole. Historically, birth was a social event that included group participation of the women in the community (Mason, 1990; Kitzinger, 1997). Perhaps in those times there was little need to express the birth story, as everyone would have known what had happened, anyway! Within western culture, where the majority of childbirth takes place in a hospital setting away from a woman's community, the need to relate the birth story may now be greater, to enable acceptance and establishment into society. According to Kirkham (1997), through telling our story we communicate our sense of self. This may be a necessary step for the woman as she assesses her new self in the light of being a mother, and establishes the subsequent changes in relationships that follow (Rubin, 1984; Raphael-Leff, 1991). Kirkham (1997) also suggests that listening to others' birth stories enables women to prepare for labour and motherhood themselves, and enables midwives to learn. Therefore, the telling of stories is a two-way process that is beneficial to the teller and the listener.

Antenatal assessment

Within the antenatal period the booking process provides an opportunity for the woman to tell her story, whether she has previously given birth or not. She may want to describe her relationships, or her working life, or within the spiritual sense may wish to establish what is meaningful to her. However, generally, the booking interview at the present time is more likely to be a question and answer session on health matters with closed questions that do not enable deeper exploration. It is argued that facilitating story-telling enables improved assessment (Burkhardt, 1994). This implies that a woman's needs would be met more effectively through this process. Such assessment may need to take place after the development of a relationship, but in present patterns of care, the woman may not have the opportunity to have such continuity.

Birth stories

Simkin's (1991) study of the long-term memories of first birth experiences demonstrated that, not only did women vividly remember their experiences, but they also wanted to retell and to relive them. For women in the pilot of a more recent study, they were unable to begin the story at the birth but had to tell the whole story of the pregnancy from the start (O'Shea, 1998). This indicates that the story of the birth has its roots in the experiences the woman has had within the pregnancy. From these studies we can establish that women appear to want to talk about their experiences. This may be as a way of making sense of them, to understand why certain things happened, or to establish the 'new self', as previously suggested. Within communities this may take place informally through toddler groups or coffee mornings. Formally, postnatal groups or postnatal listening services are available, and research has shown these to be effective for some women (Lavender and Walkinshaw, 1998). It has been implied that the retelling of stories has a healing effect (Rawlings, 1995; Taylor, 1997), which may be an argument for further encouraging the development of such services.

The process of the mother telling her story also serves to highlight the discrepancies between the official story of the experience recorded by the professionals and the perceptions of the woman concerned. This is illustrated through comparison of the authoritative language that is used and the descriptive nature of women's stories (Kirkham, 1997). The description of issues such as pain perception and provision of pain relief may provide insight into how the woman was really feeling, while the midwife's recording in the notes of the method of analgesia employed may not reveal the whole story. The telling by the woman bridges the gap and allows the midwife to understand what was important to her in the experience. In this way, the words give a sense of meaning to the experience for the woman concerned and allows the midwife a chance to grow through the hearing of such stories.

Reflection: In what ways have women described their stories to you? What language did they use in their descriptions and how was it different to the authoritative record of events?

Story-telling and the midwife

Story-telling in the provision of spiritual care could be identified in two ways:

- Through facilitation of the process in others.
- Through the carer using stories as a form of care.

As midwives are people with spiritual needs, it could be seen that story-telling may be an aspect of their own personal expression as well.

Facilitating the telling

The enabling of story-telling has been identified as an aspect of spiritual care in relation to assessment (Burkhardt, 1994; Taylor, 1997). For Taylor (1997) the encouragement of the telling will 'promote connectedness and meaningfulness'. Therefore, in the assessment process the woman may be encouraged to tell her story in such a way as to provide meaning to her previous experiences and to enable connection between herself and the listener. In being the listener, Burkhardt (1998) states that she gains insight into the person's:

- Supportive connections
- Broken relationships
- Sources of strength
- Meaningful life experiences
- Questions in respect of life's meanings.

Kirkham (1997) argues that the act of a midwife listening effectively to a woman's story will demonstrate the high value placed on her as a person and will serve to raise her self-esteem. In practice it will need time, and probably the development of a relationship, before a woman may be encouraged to share of herself in such a way.

Reflection: In what ways have you been effective in listening to a woman's story?

The process of telling may be facilitated through groups such as parenting courses, by encouraging the relating of personal stories by members to each other. This may be beneficial in enabling networking and support, but some women may find it threatening and will not wish to participate (James, 1995). Facilitation may also take place within postnatal groups or postnatal listening services (e.g. Smith and Mitchell, 1996) where women are able to relate their birth experiences to each other or to a professional. It is beneficial for midwives to be part of such groups, to enable them to see how women perceive the way they are treated in labour or their perceptions of issues such as pain and pain relief. It is argued that hearing the woman's side will enable the midwife to have a more complete picture of the birth process than would come through having just the official version of events (Kirkham, 1997). Some women have also benefited through writing down the story of the birth experience (Hebblethwaite, 1984; LaChance, 1991; Rich, 1992; Bates, 1997). Such creativity may be encouraged by a sensitive midwife to enable self-growth in the woman.

It is to be noted that recounting dreams may also be regarded as a form of spiritual story-telling. Dreams may be a way of expressing subconscious fears or anxieties, or a way of coming to terms with a change of status (Raphael-Leff, 1993). It is argued that dream-telling groups enable understanding of the dreams, providing insight into their meaning (Dombeck, 1995). It is not known how helpful such groups would be for pregnant women, but by listening and encouraging women to speak of their dreams, a midwife may assist the process of understanding and development.

> *Reflection: Is it appropriate or possible to encourage women to share their innermost feelings or dreams? Do women offer these voluntarily?*

Midwives' stories

Is it possible that stories can be used as a form of spiritual care? Taylor (1997) argues that listening to others is important, but that there may be instances where the listener may use stories to help. For instance:

- Using a story about a similar patient and how they found comfort.
- Using stories to teach about the illness or to demonstrate different attitudes to the situation.

The carer's personal story may be helpful, but Taylor (1997) warns of the motives behind the person relating the story and states that it is not appropriate for the nurse to tell the story to fulfil her own personal needs.

Case history 8

Ann was in labour with her first child on a busy labour ward. She had arrived a couple of hours ago and had been admitted into the room by a Midwifery Sister who had then rushed off to do something else. Since that time she had been 'visited' by Andrea, a staff midwife, every half hour to check she was all right and to perform various tasks to check on the baby. She was attached to a CTG to monitor the baby's heart. The contractions were becoming stronger and more uncomfortable and she had discussed with her partner, Jo, about asking for something for the pain. When Andrea came in the next time Ann told her that it was beginning to hurt. As Andrea 'did the obs', as she called it, she said: 'Well, if I were you, I would opt for an epidural now. When I had my first baby it was very painful. In fact, you are only in the early stages now and it is likely to get much worse. It would be more sensible for you to have an epidural put in now and that will keep you going. I found it wonderful – it took away all my pain and I felt great afterwards. We have the anaesthetist outside now if you want.' Ann discussed this further with Jo who suggested that it might be a good idea. As requested, the anaesthetist came in and started to put in the epidural cannula. Meanwhile the contractions had grown stronger and Ann began to complain of pressure in her back passage. The anaesthetist did not get any further, as it became obvious that Ann had progressed into the second stage of labour and she gave birth in a short time to a healthy girl.

The above story illustrates the inappropriateness of relating the midwife's own birth story and experience to the woman, rather than assessing her situation as an individual and meeting her needs. The trauma of being prepared for insertion of an epidural cannula when in labour could have been avoided.

James (1995) also warns carers of relating stories about others and the risks of gossiping or breaking codes of confidentiality. This is especially appropriate in situations on wards or in classes where women have developed relationships and then ask staff for information. Whereas sharing promotes connection and networking, the issue of confidentiality must remain paramount and requires care.

Reflection: In your experience can you think of times when stories have been related inappropriately?

Stories of experiences are also valid in the process of teaching and learning. The process of midwives sharing instances during their practice enables others to learn. However, generally midwives appear less willing to share or discuss situations, perhaps for fear of repercussions if they feel they have gone against local protocols and practices or if they have acted on instinct rather than on research evidence. In an article in the *British Journal of Midwifery* in 1996 a call was made to encourage midwives to write about critical incidents that had happened to enable a process of learning for others (Chesney, 1996). It is noticeable that there was little response following this article. The process of reflection, whether written or thought about, is valid in assisting a midwife to assess her own practice. Using these thoughts to then provide insight to others is valid and helpful as long as the codes of confidentiality are maintained. However, Kirkham (1997) suggests there has been a loss of simplicity due to the jargon that is used in writings, and that it could be argued that we should return to a more simple vocabulary to provide greater understanding to more people.

Reflection: How may midwives be encouraged to use stories as tools to enable learning and development?

Conclusion

For pregnant and postnatal women, being enabled to tell their story may be an important part of their spiritual growth. The telling may:

- Establish a woman as part of her community.
- Prepare others for labour and motherhood.
- Provide the key to appropriate care, as a form of assessment.
- Enable her to make sense of what has happened to her.
- Enable her self-growth.
- Promote healing from bad experiences.

The midwife can enable the process of story-telling through:

- Antenatal care.
- Postnatal groups and support services.
- Effective listening skills.
- Avoiding professional jargon in language, whether written or spoken.
- Enabling discussion about the woman's dreams.

This process may be best achieved through developing continuity and connection of relationship. Care should be taken in using the midwife's own stories and experiences inappropriately to manipulate others and in ensuring that confidentiality is maintained.

10 Teaching and learning spirituality in midwifery

The lack of attention to spiritual topics in the midwifery literature indicates that there is a need for spiritual awareness to be addressed within midwifery education, as it is within nursing (Burnard, 1988; Rew, 1989; Harrison *et al.*, 1993; Narayanasamy, 1993). In essence this is a difficult chapter to write, as there seem to be few answers as to 'how' the process of teaching spirituality as a subject to students should take place. It is hoped, however, that the previous chapters have demonstrated 'why' spirituality should no longer be ignored by midwife educationalists. The fact that spirituality and spiritual care is recorded as an aspect in the Midwives Rules (UKCC, 1993, p. 13) is an indication that educational institutions have a responsibility to include it within midwifery training courses. At present, there appear to be no courses in the UK where the subject is included, though sessions describing the role of the Chaplain may be addressed. It is ironic, too, that though the nursing profession is further on in their understanding of spirituality, there is still a lack of teaching within educational institutions (McSherry and Draper, 1997).

A question also remains as to whether spiritual care is something that can be taught to another or whether it is something that grows or develops within the individual. Clark *et al.* (1991) argue for the subject to be addressed in educational programmes as they believe this will help change the individuals' attitudes, knowledge and behaviours, to enable spiritual care to be effective. However, it has been demonstrated that those who give effective spiritual care have reached some personal spiritual understanding themselves (Waugh, 1992). Though training may assist those who undertake it to think about these issues if they have not done so before, it has yet to be proved that it will enable spiritual care.

Reflection: Is there room in a midwifery curriculum to introduce sessions of spiritual development? Could this be included within sessions relating to self-development and self-knowledge? Who will teach spiritual care? Must that person have reached some level of spiritual understanding themselves? Who will then judge the quality of such teaching? How can we judge/evaluate/assess students who have gone through such modules? Should we assess such a subject that is so deeply personal or ingrained?

Perhaps the issue of formal teaching is not the issue to be addressed, but instead more workshops facilitated along the lines of those used by

Burnard (1988; also see Harrison and Burnard, 1993), where the students are encouraged to explore the concepts of spirituality and its application to caring for patients. Such teaching may be more appropriate in continuing education programmes. It is also valid to recognize concerns that there is a danger of imposing the lecturer's beliefs and values on the students through this method (Bradshaw, 1997). However, this could be argued to be the case for any type of teaching method employed. Another suggestion has been for self-directed learning to be used as a method in educational programmes (Narayanasamy, 1993). If considering this method, is it enough to give students just self-directed packages to enable them to give spiritual care? Can we assume that self-development will take place?

Until there is a greater research knowledge-base for midwifery there could be an argument to ignore the teaching of spiritual issues completely. This may be a valid view in our evidence-based culture, but there are many issues that have been taught or practised clinically that have little evidence to support them. It could also be argued that there is enough evidence from the nursing literature to support the need to develop teaching methods for midwifery. With the presence now of a few taught nursing sessions, is there an argument to include midwives within these groups for the theoretical input, and use small-group, profession-specific seminars to provide the clinical information? An alternative would be to develop whole modules dedicated to spiritual issues for midwives.

Curriculum planning

If there is to be development of educational courses that include spiritual content there needs to be some understanding of why the subject has been ignored so far. It is argued (Oldnall, 1996) that educationalists:

- Are lacking in guidance and education about the value of spiritual issues to patients.
- Feel embarrassed due to spirituality not being considered scientific and being difficult to measure.

Barriers to development

A recent paper explores the issues in relation to nursing curricula and there could be a similar picture with respect to midwifery educators (McSherry and Draper, 1997). McSherry and Draper argue that spiritual issues were incorporated into programmes in the USA in 1985 but that there are barriers to this happening in the UK, from within the educational establishments themselves (intrinsic) and from the present society that exists (extrinsic).

They suggest intrinsic barriers to introducing change are:

- Hostility and opposition of educationalists.
- Having too many demands on time already.
- The need to update and develop the relevant skills and knowledge.
- The need to redesign modules.
- Change being time-consuming.
- The implications on cost and resources.
- The possible need to replace a subject with a new one.

They suggest extrinsic barriers are caused by unconsciously reflecting the present values and attitudes within our materialistic society.

Continuing education programmes

Boutell and Bozett (1990) developed an inventory to assess whether a group of American nurses assessed patients' spiritual needs effectively in order to develop an appropriate continuing education programme. This inventory asked for information on the following:

- How and to what extent nurses assessed spiritual needs.
- Indicators of spirituality used in assessment.
- Method of data collection used.
- Characteristics of nurses who assessed spirituality.

From this they suggested that a programme should include:

- Basic knowledge of spirituality.
- Nursing assessment and interventions.
- Values and spiritual needs.
- The importance of spiritual dimensions of human experience to nursing practice.
- Teaching by clergy about specific religions.

Boutell and Bozett highlight that teaching the theory of spirituality is not enough and further recommend using clinical experiences and demonstrating spiritual assessments as the basis for discussions in the classroom. Though this is primarily a plan for the continuing education of qualified nurses, such a plan may be adapted for use with pre-registration courses.

Nursing process model

Ross (1996) proposes using a framework based on the nursing process as a way of providing spiritual care, from which she suggests a teaching plan can be developed. She highlights the need to include:

- Teaching regarding broad theories about spirituality.
- Awareness of spiritual needs.
- Recognition of the nurses' limitations and referral to others.

Though the nursing process as a form of assessment has been in use some time, there remains a question as to its validity in midwifery, and therefore such teaching will have limitations in training midwifery students.

Developing intuition

Rew (1989) has argued for educationalists to address intuitive practice within programmes. She states that there is a need to:

- Clarify the concepts of intuition and spirituality.
- Address the subject in educational programmes.
- Teach students how to assess from cues given and interpret them in order to be able to judge clinically.
- Value intuition and analytical thinking in students as complementary to other skills.
- Encourage the documenting of how nurses make decisions, therefore increasing understanding of intuitive processes.

Her paper then describes exercises that could be used as tools to enhance a person's intuition and spiritual growth. Though this method may be used as a tool to aid in developing decision-making generally, it could also be regarded as appropriate in a programme relating to spiritual issues, but would need further adaptation to be used within the context of midwifery.

Guidelines to spiritual care

Within a paper dealing with addressing needs in relation to spiritual distress, the author gives guidelines to enable nurses provide spiritual care (Sumner, 1998). These are:

- Help the person find meaning and purpose in life. Try to understand her individual way of experience and expression of her spirituality. Encourage her to review her life so far and listen carefully to her.
- Be completely 'present and open' to situations that arise when interacting with the patient.
- Be aware of different religions and other practices relating to a person's faith. Provide the environment and space for her ritual and devotional practices.
- Use direct questioning about spiritual issues. Use answers to plan effective interventions of care.

- Be trustworthy and accepting.
- Help the person in developing her spiritual side.
- Be aware of others in the health care team to whom you may refer.
- Be aware of a person's spiritual supporters and aim to work with them.

These guidelines are broad enough to provide a framework from which practical educational sessions on the role of the midwife could be adapted.

Proposed framework for teaching

As these papers have illustrated, there are few educational programmes in use at the present time that could be adapted for the purposes of delivering programmes to midwifery students. Therefore there is a need to develop something completely new. To this end the following subjects are proposed, which could be used in a module for teaching spirituality and spiritual issues to midwives:

---

1. Theory of spirituality and spiritual care.
2. Cultural/religious spiritual needs – including specific clinical needs and influences on choices.
3. Relationships: fostering a culture of understanding; changes in the woman's life.
4. Effective assessment, including listening skills and story-telling.
5. The development of self: the woman during pregnancy and the midwife.
6. Intuitive skills.
7. Spiritual needs of those without specific religious beliefs.
8. Spirituality and the organization of care.
9. Awareness of local spiritual support networks.
10. Role of religious carers in midwifery support.
11. Spiritual issues surrounding the unborn baby.
12. Fostering a spiritual environment.
13. Teaching spirituality in parenting courses.

Though untested at the present time, this framework contains the elements that are included within nursing programmes and adapts them to the needs of the student midwife, and could be developed within any midwifery programme. Theoretical assessment could be carried out through assignments, but it would also be desirable to have assessment within the clinical setting. Ideally the two strands of assessment could be linked to ensure linking theory to practice.

Some would argue that the subject should be taught integrally or holistically across the board within other midwifery areas. This may be valid; however, as the subject is not being addressed at all at the present time, there needs to be a firm decision to include spiritual issues within a programme, ensuring that all the relevant aspects are covered and evaluated, before including the subject with anything else. Certainly, with time, issues relating to the baby and motherhood could become part of sessions dealing with postnatal care, and others, such as self-development or spiritual networks, part of sessions on labour or antenatal care. Inclusion of other spiritual carers, such as Chaplains, will enable greater understanding of their role. It may well take some time and effort to have such a module accepted as part of a midwifery programme. It may also be the case that such developments will be more closely evaluated by peers than other programmes, due to the generally unacceptable material that will be produced!

Parenthood education

The last aspect of the proposed teaching framework mentions the aspects of teaching spirituality on parenting courses. At the present time there are no professional bodies running formal preparation classes for parenting within the UK that actively include spirituality. However, it is necessary to state that there are specific parenting courses or self-help groups run by women that do address spirituality (e.g. Stockley, 1986). The use of certain relaxation techniques such as yoga has spiritual undertones and it is necessary to be aware of those women who have explored such methods to a greater depth and intensity than just for exercise. In the USA, midwives such as those at The Farm community address spirituality as a way of life, with the expectation that pregnant women will do the same (Gaskin, 1977). Also church organizations such as the Australian Childbirth and Parenting Ministries (Childbirth and Parenting Ministries, 1999) may approach preparation for parenting from a specifically religious perspective. From this it could be ascertained that midwives:

- Should be aware of the types of parenting groups available locally.
- Should be aware of the groups the women in their care are attending or have attended.
- May be involved in setting up programmes that approach the subject of spirituality for childbirth and parenting.

Conclusion

Within the UK at the present time there is little to offer students on midwifery programmes in terms of development or understanding of spiritual issues. In this chapter, some of the papers that have been written describing the development of spirituality in nursing programmes have been investigated, and an attempt has been made to develop a programme that could be offered to teach the subject to midwives or students. Further, an attempt has been made at describing parenting teaching on offer at the moment that addresses spiritual issues. Such a chapter has limitations and over time it is hoped that programmes will be developed that will grow understanding and enable midwives to provide spiritual care as an integral part of their practice.

11 *Midwifery spiritual care: working with others*

Health professionals do not work in a vacuum and midwives are not an exception. Daily in the practical work they undertake, whether community or hospital based, they need to link and communicate with others from associated health professions. There is also a need for midwives to work with women and their lay carers. Up to now this book has focussed on the potential spiritual role for midwives, but it is also appropriate to address the role of others who may provide spiritual support or care to pregnant women and their families.

> *Reflection: Have you had contact with people who provide spiritual support to pregnant women? In your opinion has this support been of value to the woman concerned? Did it appear to meet her needs at that time?*

Discussion about the subject matter of this book with midwives has revealed that many believe spiritual care is not within their remit but should be the province of religious ministers alone. Narayanasamy (1993) argues that this need to depend on religious ministers to provide care is a method nurses use to avoid getting involved in giving spiritual care themselves. As already indicated, this also avoids discussion of the role of the midwife in spiritual care currently assumed in the present rules of practice (UKCC, 1993). This belief that spiritual care is someone else's role assumes that:

- All women have a religious belief that has a corresponding minister who can provide care.
- Ministers will be available to provide care at the time it is required.
- All religious ministers are able or want to give spiritual care within maternity settings.

The ability to provide ministry is further complicated by the fact that in many structured religions the ministers are often male. For some women the issues of reproduction and childbirth are culturally and personally 'women's work' and the thought of consulting a male minister would be abhorrent. There may also be a suggestion that a woman who has given birth herself may be a better person to provide spiritual care than a minister who has no understanding of the experience of childbirth and motherhood.

Reflection: Do you believe spiritual care should only be given by religious ministers? Do you think the fact that many religious ministers are male is a problem in giving care in maternity settings?

A woman may gain spiritual support from a variety of sources. In a study of how patients with cancer use strategies for coping with their illness it was shown that the patients generally relied on a combination of people to provide spiritual support (Sodestrom and Martinson, 1987). Some of the study population thought staff had too little time for spiritual matters and, therefore, help was mostly sought from family, clergy and friends, with only a few asking for help from nurses and physicians. Within maternity settings, women may gain strength from others such as:

- Local ministers of religion
- Spiritual mentors
- Hospital chaplains
- Their partners
- Friends and family.

The midwife would need to be aware of these sources of support and know how to contact them should the need arise. Each of these sources may have particular roles to play within the woman's pregnancy and within the postnatal period. The rest of this chapter will focus upon these potential roles and the relationship with midwifery care. However, as ministers of some religions do not have a pastoral role within their communities, the descriptions of professional spiritual leaders have been limited mainly to those of mainstream religious ministers in the UK. For investigation of the roles of those of other beliefs and countries it would be beneficial to look at other sources.

Local ministers

In previous chapters it has been mentioned that historically the relationship between midwives and ministers of various organized religions has not always been a good one. The 'wise woman' role of midwives was often regarded as a threat to the male authority in churches and medicine, with the result that some midwives were regarded as witches within certain communities (Achterberg, 1990). More recently in the UK there has been little interconnection between religious ministers and community health care workers, unless the minister has a particular interest in aspects of health.

Reflection: In your opinion should there be some effort at communication between primary health workers and local religious leaders? Who should be responsible for instigating this process?

Communication issues

In our present culture of developing holistic care and increased openness to different approaches to health care it would be appropriate to improve the communication between those primarily associated with provision of physical care and those primarily involved in spiritual care. Some of the difficulties associated with past relationships are related to a lack of understanding of each other's roles and responsibilities. It is worth noting that, in many ways, these roles overlap with each other.

Another difficulty in the development of this relationship is the assumption by many health care workers that those being cared for do not want the involvement of specific spiritual carers unless they ask for it. However, in a study of patients' attitudes to medical referral for spiritual care, the finding that was most constant was that doctors should refer patients to clergy or professionals trained in spiritual care if there was a perceived spiritual problem (Daaleman and Nease, 1994). The same authors mention a further study of general practitioners' attitudes, where referral to clergy was dependent on:

- The physician's religious belief or lack of it.
- The need for the right clergy to be available.
- The assumption that the religious patient would self-refer and that the non-religious patient would not want referral.
- Lack of knowledge about the role of the clergy in clinical practice (Jones, 1990).

It is probable that such attitudes would be prevalent among any health care workers, including midwives. In a study looking at the relationship between nurses and chaplains (VandeCreek, 1997), it is further indicated that patients want the involvement of parish clergy in their spiritual care. Here 60 per cent of the patients studied identified a community clergy member they would contact for support. The author suggests the need for collaboration with these clergy, especially as they had been selected by the patient as their support. Communication between hospital staff and chaplains and the patient's own minister is an issue, especially in situations where patients are constantly in and out of hospital (Keighley, 1997). In midwifery terms this situation may not arise often, except where women have particular antenatal problems that require frequent admissions for tests or medical care. However, the need for effective communication is appropriate if the woman wants to maintain the supportive relationship with her local minister. How this triad of communication is to take place and with whom the responsibility lies is yet to be effectively explored.

In order to improve communication and understanding of roles it is viewed that midwives would benefit from knowing the community structure in which they are located and being aware of the possible sources of support that are available (Corrine and Bailey, 1992). This may include awareness of religious groups that have sources of support for women during pregnancy or postnatally. Though it would be impossible to expect every midwife to personally know every minister of every religious persuasion within her working area, links could be attempted through attendance of meetings relating to health, or specifically maternity care, where understanding could be developed.

Reflection: Are you aware of the community in which you work and the sources from which women gain spiritual support? How could you find out about these sources and disseminate the information to colleagues?

Involvement in pregnancy

Over history there has generally been little involvement of local ministers during the time of a woman's normal pregnancy, unless she particularly chooses to ask for support or prayer. A large majority of women do not reveal their pregnancy until it begins to 'show' or until after antenatal test results are known or until the risk of losing the pregnancy by a miscarriage has passed. This is often the time when women experience some of the unpleasant side effects of early pregnancy, such as nausea, vomiting, tiredness or urinary frequency. As a result they may not attend usual religious meetings, if they have a belief, or may isolate themselves from the local community. It would be unusual to expect involvement in care by local ministers during this time.

However, there is evidence to suggest that women do turn to ministers in times of difficulty or conflict during pregnancy. For instance, some women turn to religious ministers to provide advice and support over decisions relating to termination of the pregnancy, and it has been recorded that women turn to them for counsel after terminations have taken place (Marck, 1994). Sowell and Misener's study (1997) of the decision making of women infected with HIV on whether to keep or terminate their pregnancies, showed that some women were influenced in their decisions by ministers and religious teachings. These authors suggest that HIV education should be encouraged within church communities, as 'religious groups may have an unparalleled opportunity to provide comfort and assistance to women in making important life decisions' (p. 68). Other women have been known to ask for help on issues relating to difficulties with fertility and decisions relating to suspected abnormality of the fetus.

Case history 9

Hannah, at 35 years old, was expecting her first baby. She had already met her local midwife, Jill, who had carried out blood tests, including screening tests for the fetal abnormalities of Down's syndrome and spina bifida at Hannah's request. An ultrasound scan was also booked at the local hospital for when the pregnancy had reached 19 weeks. However, before Hannah reached that time Jill called to tell her that the screening test showed that the risk of the baby having Down's syndrome was high. Hannah was very upset and Jill spent time with her explaining the options open to her. Leaving Hannah written information about the results, Jill returned later when Hannah's partner, Steve, came home from work. She then explained the situation again, to them both this time. At this point Hannah revealed that, as a child, she had attended a church school and now found it difficult to make a decision about terminating a pregnancy. Jill suggested the couple talk the issues over with their local minister, but Hannah indicated that until that time they had chosen not to have contact with the church. As Jill had recently attended an infant baptism at the church she offered to contact the minister and ask him to talk through the issues with them. Hannah and Steve were grateful for the offer and subsequently received a home visit from the minister, who discussed the potential issues with them both. He offered to pray for them and, though they did not join in, they were thankful for the suggestion. When the time came for the diagnostic tests the minister promised to be offering prayer support for them and made himself available to be contacted by them if required. The tests were able to show that Hannah was carrying a normal pregnancy, which continued successfully to the birth of a normal girl. Hannah and Steve were grateful for the intervention and support of both the midwife and minister and subsequently asked him to baptise their daughter as a way of saying thank you to him.

Reflection: In this story the midwife instigated contact with the minister. Do you believe this was an appropriate action on her part or do you believe it should have been left to the couple to make contact? Would you have acted in the same way?

In the above case the minister was able to give the necessary support to the couple involved. However, for a religious minister to be able to provide appropriate spiritual advice he would need to have intimate knowledge and understanding of pregnancy, the issues relating to fetal testing and abnormality and the experiences that a woman and her partner will be going through. It is to be debated as to whether religious ministers of any kind are equipped to do this work. To enable this development it may be appropriate to set up community based groups where midwives, other community health carers and religious leaders could forge links and provide mutual support in giving care. There could also be situations where midwives could be involved in teaching on courses for religious leaders to enable an exchange of knowledge to take place.

Reflection: Do you believe it is realistic to include local religious leaders in the primary health care team?

Involvement in labour

Generally, it is unusual to have involvement of religious ministers in labour care. However, there are situations where they may be present in the home or a maternity unit if they are personal friends of the woman in labour or where they have been involved in care during the antenatal period. This may be particularly relevant if there is known to be abnormality or illness within this or a previous pregnancy, and the woman or her partner have asked for support. If the minister is present the midwife should be aware of how the woman wishes him or her to be included within the labour. Care should be taken about maintaining confidentiality but also ensuring that the woman receives the spiritual support she requires.

Reflection: How would you feel as a midwife if a woman requested the presence of her local religious minister during her labour? How would you approach the situation?

In some situations the minister's role in labour care may be to pray for the woman and her partner as she is going through the experience. In some areas couples will have set up a 'prayer network' – a group of believers of the same religion who are praying for the couple and unborn child – and the minister will be the link to this network. It is common for this to have been set up prior to attendance by a midwife and she may be unaware of this taking place unless the minister requests information on progress via the telephone. It is essential that no confidential information is given unless it is at the request of the couple concerned.

Involvement postnatally

As discussed in previous chapters, for a woman with belief there may be an increase in religious activities following the birth of her baby. This may include specific rituals associated with her religion, with the purpose of 'welcoming' the new child or addressing the 'rite of passage' the woman herself has experienced. A local minister of religion may or may not be involved in such rituals, especially in societies where the woman may be regarded as 'impure' or 'unclean' if she is still losing blood vaginally. In some situations women will actively seek religion after the birth of their new baby, especially if they have had links with this religion in the past within their family.

In the UK Christian tradition, where there has been a birth a local minister may pastorally visit the new infant and parents at home if they are aware of the family or have had some involvement within the antenatal period. Their role may be to 'welcome' the new life through prayer. For some it may be to act as a link with other members of the church community and to initiate practical support following assessment of need at that visit.

Case history 10

One religious community the author is aware of sets up a team of people who are able to provide practical support following the birth of a baby. For example, this may be through providing childcare for other children, cleaning services and/or hot meals every night for a week. If the new parents have family support the church community help is initiated when the family support runs out. This assessment of need may be carried out by the minister himself or delegated to another person who is able to fulfil that role.

In these situations the minister will need to be informed about the arrival of the new child in order to carry out such visits. This may be done by the new parents themselves or through being informed by members of the local community. For some this may seem like an intrusion, and it is appropriate to ensure that the family wants this kind of practical support before it is given. A midwife may not be involved in such care but should be aware if local churches are offering this kind of postnatal service in case they are asked about it by new parents.

> *Reflection: Are you aware of what kind of practical support is offered in your community to new parents through local churches?*

Other communities may provide support through the provision of baby equipment to those in need and many have women's groups specifically aimed at providing a place where women can get out of the home and develop friendships. Some of these have particular times that are geared to giving health education advice or information, and midwives and health visitors may be asked to be involved in such sessions. These situations may be ideal opportunities to develop links with local church communities.

Some women may turn to religion for support and comfort in instances where the birth has not been as expected. For example, some women turned to religion in a study of mothers of preterm babies (Brady-Fryer, 1994). Local ministers may be involved in providing counsel and support to such women and their families, and in situations where the child has been born with an abnormality. In these situations, again, it may be difficult for a minister to provide effective care and help to women in need of spiritual support without the necessary knowledge and information. As described in the section relating to antenatal care, a local midwife may be able to be a source of the appropriate information, but care must again be taken to pay attention to confidentiality and whether the parents are wanting the involvement of the minister.

Reflection: In your experience, do women turn to religion after the birth of their babies? Do you know how local ministers in your area provide postnatal support to women who have had problems following the birth of a child?

Circumcision

Some religions and cultures require boy infants to be circumcised. For Jewish families this will be around the eighth day after birth. For Islamic families it could be within the early days after birth, though it can wait until later, as long as it is before the boy reaches puberty. Though it is uncommon for this to take place in hospital involving a religious leader facilities should be in place in case a family requires it before the infant goes home. However, for any midwives providing postnatal care there needs to be awareness of when this may take place in order to appropriately observe the child.

Midwifery support

In situations where a midwife has a belief she may also receive support in her work from her local minister. In some areas this may be through specific worship services that are geared to highlighting and praying for the work of health care workers. In other situations it may be through the midwife setting up a network of mutual believers to provide prayer support during her daily work (Davis, 1996). She may then call on this network in times of crisis to pray for specific situations. A local minister may or may not be involved in such a network. However, the midwife may also call upon a minister to provide moral or ethical guidance in situations where she is experiencing conflict between her beliefs and the situation in which she is working. Care must be taken to maintain confidentiality in such times of counsel, especially if they relate to particular cases.

Reflection: Have there been times in your practice when you would have welcomed the opportunity to discuss moral or ethical issues with an 'outsider'? Have you ever thought of turning to a religious minister for this?

Spiritual mentors

In previous chapters it has been described how women with or without religious belief may find sources of spiritual support and care from others outside the family circle. Religious ministers may fulfil this role, as already described above, or there may be others who could be regarded as a woman's spiritual mentor. Such contacts may be made in relation to active participation in political or social groups. For pregnant women, joining a specific birth group or antenatal class, such as those run by the National Childbirth Trust, may serve to meet spiritual needs.

Reflection: Are you aware of women in your care who receive what could be regarded as spiritual support from sources other than religious ministers?

Communication issues

In order to provide effective spiritual care a midwife will need to be aware of sources of support and know what women want from carers. This is certainly easier where continuity of care is practised and the midwife has been able to develop a relationship with the women in her care. It is important for the midwife to understand and have intimate knowledge of the information, support and experience women receive from antenatal groups they attend. As with the available support from religious ministers, it may be unrealistic for every midwife to know every potential supportive group. However, when a midwife becomes aware of a woman's attendance at a group, efforts could be made to establish a link at that time for the sake of the individual care of the woman concerned. It may be helpful, therefore, for a midwife to attend the groups and find out what women are being told, and then to develop ways of working with them. Ways of establishing relationships with leaders of these groups should be found in order to foster a mutual understanding of roles.

Reflection: Are you aware of the information women are being given in local antenatal support groups? Have you attended any?

Involvement in the antenatal period

A woman may turn to others in pregnancy to enable her to find understanding and support for the experiences she is going through. The connecting relationship that sometimes develops between midwife and woman could be regarded as spiritual, and women may rely on the midwife to fulfil this role. Others may experience this support through relationships developed in antenatal groups.

Stockley (1986) describes her involvement with a birth group intent on providing spiritual support and a place where women were able to stop and get in touch with their unborn baby spiritually. Her belief is that 'spiritual nutrition' is as important as 'biological nutrition' for the unborn baby's growth and development. The group also encourages women to respond intuitively to their unborn baby and the pregnancy and to recognise where there may be potential problems. Stockley views that 'parents are experts just as much as doctors'. It is this latter attitude that has caused most disquiet among some health carers over the years when dealing with women who have attended such support groups. Some women will turn to their mentor rather than midwife for information about specific issues of antenatal care, or will ask the mentor to reiterate information the midwife has supplied. A spiritual mentor may also attend antenatal appointments with the woman concerned if a problem is anticipated, especially in situations where there is perceived to be conflict with medical advisors. In effect, the mentor is acting as an advocate. It is understandable that some midwives have found such approaches to be threatening to their practice. Improved communication between carers and understanding of the information given by each other would assist in resolving conflict and enable working together in order to meet a woman's needs.

> *Reflection: Have you been in a situation where a woman has brought someone with her to an appointment to ask questions for her or to act as a prompt for her own questioning? Did you welcome the person being there or did you find this experience threatening? How did you deal with your feelings?*

Involvement during labour

Following the antenatal support that a spiritual mentor will have provided the woman may then request the mentor to be a birth supporter. Their role may be to act as an instructor of pain relieving techniques taught in antenatal classes, to be a 'spiritual advisor', and may also to be an advocate for the woman or couple during the process of labour. In these situations some midwives have felt threatened in their practise, especially if they have had no knowledge of the content of the classes the woman has attended or if they have not been involved with the mentor before. Once more, the need for midwives to be aware of the kind of support women receive in their locality is vital to giving appropriate care. Such situations are better managed in the woman's own environment and where the midwife has been able to get to know the woman, and possibly her mentor, prior to labour. It is beneficial to have knowledge of the mentor, to enable a positive relationship to develop, and for trust and understanding, so that the woman will receive the most appropriate support from all concerned.

Reflection: Have you been present at a birth where a woman has brought an antenatal supporter or spiritual advisor with her? How did you react in this situation and what was their role in the labour?

Postnatal involvement

It is common for women who have been actively involved in antenatal support groups to want to continue these after the baby has been born. These links provide strong bonds of friendship between women, but may also enable mutual teaching of developing motherhood skills, and encourage spiritual growth and development of both the woman and her child. Groups may encourage support through mentoring programmes – a new mother being supported by another more experienced. Information about baby care and feeding skills also serve to enable the woman to grow as a mother. Lay breastfeeding counsellors have evolved over a time where midwives' skills have been more concentrated on pregnancy and labour, but frequently midwives have felt undermined by their presence. More recently their value is being recognised and midwives are encouraging women to contact such supporters for help and advice. This has been enabled by improved communication and understanding of each others' roles, as well as recognising the worth of skilled women who have trained specifically to give breastfeeding advice.

Reflection: Are you aware of the types of postnatal support that are available to women in your locality? Apart from feeding, in what other ways are women given support? Do you feel this should be the role of the midwife?

Hospital chaplains

Within the UK, hospital trusts may employ the services of chaplains to fulfil a spiritual role. These may be full- or part-time workers, paid or unpaid. Usually chaplaincies would have ministers from the Anglican and the Roman Catholic churches with further support from other

Christian denominations and other religions where leaders have a pastoral role. The aim is for chaplaincies to be 'multi-faith' in their outlook, but it is to be debated as to what this actually means in practical terms. There has been a long history of chaplains' involvement in health care, but there remains a lack of understanding of roles and communication between them and health care staff. Their role may be dependent on the particular trust in which they are employed. Commonly it may include administration of religious rites, dealing specifically with dying patients and their relatives, and caring for staff. Some chaplains may be on committees particularly involved with ethical considerations. As indicated in earlier chapters, there is an expectation from health care staff that it is the role of the chaplains to give spiritual care to all who need it, despite it being unrealistic to expect an individual chaplain to be available to everyone all the time (Ross, 1997). In a discussion between members of the caring professions, a chaplain stated how he identifies a 'divine spark' in everyone with whom he has contact (Savett, 1997). From this he recognises that others are also in a position to address spiritual care apart from him. However, though viewing the responsibility of spiritual care as being shared, over half of the nurses in Ross' study preferred to refer these issues mainly to the ordained clergy, rather than dealing with the circumstances themselves.

From the patient's perspective the chaplain may or may not be the most appropriate person to meet their spiritual needs. According to Ross (1997) the best person to give spiritual care should be 'anyone whom the patient trusts, has built up rapport with and, who the patient perceives, has the time'. The time issue is important in that chaplains generally have responsibility for a large hospital population and need to assess the places of greatest need. If chaplains are so stretched for time, the nurse or midwife caring for the patient may be the most appropriate person to address the spiritual need immediately, rather than having to wait for the ministrations of the chaplain.

Negatively, there has been criticism of the work of hospital chaplains, with the suggestion that, even if the patient has a different belief system to their own, the process of understanding and acknowledgement will be used to push the person into 'a "convenient" religious framework' (Edassery and Kuttierath, 1998). This criticism could be levelled at any person brought up in a religious or cultural framework where there is a desire to fit others into a particular mould of understanding. Some denominations have also been accused of bias in the way that spiritual care is offered to some but not to others (Keighley, 1997). It is clear that chaplaincy care is not viewed as perfect and there is a need to approach the issues involved in a more multidisciplinary way.

The role of the chaplain is not limited to caring for patients. In the development of a framework of practice for chaplaincy and health care staff, one chaplain indicated that over 60 per cent of his time was spent with staff (Keighley, 1997). For some, the chaplain's area of work is viewed as the 'church' with the staff members as the 'congregation' (Burke and Matsumoto, 1999). This could involve discussion about the care of particular patients but could also involve supporting staff with difficult situations concerning the type of care given or issues relating to death and dying. Burke and Matsumoto (1999) suggest that the chaplain being present may also have the effect of influencing staff to think about their own beliefs and values. They suggest that the roles of the chaplain may be:

- A creator of meaning to issues and events.
- A trustworthy listener.
- A pastor away from home.
- A calming presence.
- Someone to come alongside during grief and bereavement.
- A trigger to discuss ethical issues.
- An educator.

The accessibility of chaplains and their personality may both play a part in how able to approach them staff feel, to discuss issues that to some may feel personal. The methods of communication and abilities in communication between staff and chaplains are therefore to be regarded as important, to enable appropriate spiritual care to be given to patients and to meet the needs of the staff caring for them.

Reflection: In what ways has your current experience of working with chaplains been positive or negative? How would you aim to improve this situation?

Communication issues

Effective communication between all health carers is key to enable the needs of a particular client to be met in an appropriate way. This involves giving and receiving information in many forms, as well as the availability and accessibility of carers to discuss particular issues. Unfortunately, there remains an *ad hoc* approach to communication with chaplains by hospital midwifery staff.

From her own practice, the author has been aware of chaplains who had particular times or days when they would do 'rounds' of the wards to discover if there was anyone who needed help. Sometimes a midwife, if not too busy, would go round the clients present and ask them if they wished to talk to the chaplain. This was not a popular task and often the minister would be pointed to the Kardex and advised to look himself for potential clients! Such an approach is limiting, firstly because the staff view the 'round' as a task without much meaning, and secondly because just looking through the Kardex for clients of a particular religion may miss out others who have a spiritual need at that time.

An alternative approach is for the chaplain to only appear if contacted by the midwife. A criticism of this approach could be that some midwives would never contact the chaplain at all while others would do so all the time. This would mean some clients could receive care while others would miss out on the days certain carers were on duty. VandeCreek (1997) states that chaplains frequently rely on the referral of patients by nurses. He suggests this process is influenced by:

- Clinical assessment of need.
- A nurse's experience of and assumptions about the role and importance of religion, spirituality, pastoral care, the clergy in general and the chaplain involved.
- The individual nurse's stance in any of these matters.

VandeCreek states that chaplains 'find it helpful to know the religious and spiritual beliefs, practices and idiosyncrasies of nurses with whom they work', as this enables them to put into context the referrals they receive from individual nurses. Such information could only be gathered over time due to the limited period chaplains are able to spend in the ward area and the use of shifts by staff. It would take some effort for a chaplain to get to know each midwife's personal belief system well enough to be able to use the information appropriately.

> *Reflection: In your experience, how do chaplains receive information about the needs of particular clients? Do they just turn up or are they called? Are you proactive in calling them or do you leave this to other carers?*

In Ross' (1994) study of the factors associated with nurses giving spiritual care, those who responded suggested their ability to give spiritual care was hindered by:

- Religious ministers not being available.
- The nurse's perception that the ministers had not performed their job properly.
- A perceived lack of communication between the disciplines.

This study suggests a need for greater collaboration, as does Dombeck (1998) who addresses the need for an interprofessional approach to care. Murray and Zentner (1989) also suggest the need for a team approach to care, with an improved understanding of each other's roles and responsibilities and better communication. Nurses may include other professions within a team approach to giving care, but at the present time it is unusual for a chaplain to be involved. For the effective inclusion of a chaplain in all aspects of health care planning to occur, a greater number would need to be employed to cover the work in large hospitals. It could also be argued that it would be inappropriate to use one chaplain from a particular religion when so many clients have different beliefs.

It is to be argued from the above information that there needs to be an improvement in methods of communication between nursing staff and chaplains. Ross (1997) suggests the following to be helpful in improving collaboration:

- Maintain a list of clergy telephone numbers and times of 'on-call' availability.
- Improved communication with clergy and discussion with them as they leave and enter the ward about certain patients.
- Inclusion of clergy in ward planning or patient profile discussions, to involve him/her as a valuable member of the health care team.

Improvement in telecommunications in recent years has meant most on-call chaplains carry pagers or mobile telephones to improve accessibility. But this is of no help if the numbers to be called are not easily available to staff on duty. Knowing when chaplaincy staff are to visit the ward area is helpful, as planning can occur as to which clients need to be discussed or need pastoral care. Also, if appropriate assessment has shown that a client has a particular religious need, the chaplain or appropriate religious leader may be contacted to discuss how this need can be met. It is also recommended that any visit from a minister be recorded in the client's records (Murray and Zentner, 1989). Such steps will indicate to other members of staff the value of spiritual care and help, so that the best care can be given to clients.

> *Reflection: Do you believe the above methods of communication are appropriate or unrealistic? Do you think it is necessary to include chaplains in care planning or should they be contacted only as required?*

Involvement in the antenatal period

In UK hospitals at the present time it is unusual for a hospital chaplain to be involved in the antenatal care of a woman. Prior to the involvement of the midwife, chaplains may be active in meeting the needs of women who have suffered early pregnancy loss. This may involve assistance in arranging a burial or cremation of the infant and the provision of a service. Some chaplaincies also hold books of remembrance where the names of lost infants may be recorded as a memorial. With most care in pregnancy being carried out within the community, there may be more contact with a woman's local religious minister, as indicated above. However, in certain circumstances a midwife may recognise the need to contact a hospital chaplain for support or for assistance with the provision of spiritual care.

A midwife working in an hospital antenatal clinic may feel it appropriate to contact a chaplain if a diagnosis has been made of an abnormality within the pregnancy, especially relating to a death or extreme illness. As this will usually be after an ultrasound scan, there may be a problem with a chaplain's involvement due to the urgency of the potential crisis and the need for immediate availability. Within these situations it may be more appropriate for a midwife to provide initial spiritual support. It needs to be remembered that it should be the woman's choice as to whether a chaplain or minister of religion is to be contacted for her, rather than making an assumption that she requires this kind of help. However, a chaplain may also be helpful in providing support to relatives or members of staff dealing with these and other difficult situations, and it may be appropriate to contact the chaplain for these reasons even if the woman does not require his support. In the section relating to community ministers, the need for them to have an intimate knowledge of antenatal abnormality is discussed, in order to ensure that appropriate counsel is given. This would also apply to hospital chaplains, and a mechanism for briefing and mutual information exchange could be developed to improve spiritual care for women.

Reflection: Have there been situations in an antenatal clinic when you would have welcomed the presence of a hospital chaplain to provide spiritual care to a woman or her relatives?

On other occasions a chaplain may be involved in the antenatal care of a woman where he has had contact with her in a previous difficult pregnancy or illness. In these situations the woman herself may have requested his involvement. The midwife caring for her will need to be aware of this request and be sensitive to what the woman wants. This is especially relevant in relation to confidentiality of information and how much the woman wishes to be relayed to the chaplain. Some women with a particular religious belief may ask for a chaplain to help with making certain moral or ethical decisions related to the pregnancy. Effective briefing will again be required by the chaplain to ensure that he has understanding of the situation involved.

Reflection: Have you been aware of situations where women or their partners have requested the presence of a chaplain to aid them in their decision making? Has this been easily facilitated?

Occasionally a woman will need to spend some time being cared for in hospital for part of her pregnancy, though this is avoided as much as possible with the current use of day care facilities in some areas. However, it is during this time that a chaplain may become involved in providing pastoral care, especially if it is thought that the outcome of the pregnancy may not be good.

Case history 11

Isabelle was admitted to the antenatal ward when she was 32 weeks into a triplet pregnancy. She was feeling very tired and heavy but there were also signs of polyhydramnios and there was a suspicion that one of the babies had not been growing as well as the other two. During her admission history she indicated her involvement with a church and the midwife offered to contact the hospital chaplain for her. Isabelle said she would be pleased to meet him, and he came the next morning. He spent some time with her, which was possible as she had been given a single room, and offered to bring her Holy Communion. This became a weekly occurrence during her time in hospital and the chaplain was able to pray with both Isabelle and her husband as they prepared for the births of their children. As the pregnancy continued it became more obvious that one of the triplets was not thriving and a decision was made when the pregnancy had reached 36 weeks' gestation to deliver the babies by caesarean section. On the morning of the operation the chaplain made himself available to Isabelle and spent some time with her husband. He also waited on the labour ward until the babies had been delivered. As suspected, one of the infants, Emily, was discovered to have a serious abnormality. All of the babies were admitted initially to the special care unit and Isabelle and her husband continued to receive support from the chaplain. Sadly, a few days later, it became obvious that Emily was not going to survive, and the chaplain baptised her with both her parents present. He was available to them as the baby died and then was also able to be helpful in supporting them in the funeral arrangements. Later they requested that he take part in the service of thanksgiving that subsequently took place in their local church.

The above situation shows the value of the chaplain being able to provide long-term support into the postnatal period because of the extended admission of the woman involved. Though this situation is unusual, a chaplain may also provide such support to women who are admitted for only a short time before the birth. It is therefore appropriate for a midwife admitting a woman to be an inpatient in hospital to ask if a visit from the chaplain would be helpful to her.

Reflection: Have you been involved in a situation where a hospital chaplain has been able to provide extended support to a woman and her family in this way?

Involvement in labour

It is generally unusual for a hospital chaplain to be physically present at the birth of a child, unless it has been the specific request of the family concerned. However, there are situations where a chaplain may be available for prayer or counsel in the labour ward area, as in the illustration used above. Midwives tend to call chaplains where it is known that there is a fetal abnormality not thought to be compatible with life. A chaplain may also be available where an infant has already died in utero or where a fresh stillbirth occurs. In any situations where death is involved it is important for the midwife to be very sensitive to the couple's needs and requests and to maintain confidentiality. In a paper about stillbirth, Thomson (1981) discusses the issue of women who are not religious being grateful for any support that is offered but being reluctant to have a chaplain called in specially for that purpose. She states that the presence of a chaplain who 'just happens to be in the building' is to be viewed as an asset. It is clear too that assumptions should not be made about women's religious beliefs and there needs to be understanding of how deaths should be handled for those who do not have a Christian belief (Schott and Henley, 1996). In these tragic situations the chaplain can also be of support to staff having to deal with the grieving couple.

Case history 12

A woman was admitted into the labour unit of a large hospital. The labour progressed very slowly and the woman required an epidural for pain relief before a decision was taken to commence a Syntocinon infusion to accelerate the labour. After some hours it became apparent that the woman's cervix was fully dilated and that the baby could be born. The woman involved was exhausted by this time and was unable to push the baby out. The Registrar on duty recommended that a Ventouse delivery be carried out by the new SHO with his support, and the woman was prepared for an operative delivery. Meanwhile the heartbeat of the unborn infant remained steady. A number of attempts were made to deliver the infant's head with the Ventouse by the SHO, but little progress was made. The Registrar then recommended the use of forceps and he discovered on vaginal examination that the infant was lying in a transverse position and was not rotating easily. He applied rotational forceps, turned the infant and then proceeded to support the SHO in delivering the head at the perineum. The delivery was very difficult and it became obvious that the baby was larger than had previously been anticipated and the cord was felt to be tight around the baby's neck. It then took some time to deliver the shoulders and the rest of the child's body. At birth the infant had no heartbeat and made no respiratory effort, and though resuscitation was attempted by a paediatrician, the baby did not survive. The chaplain became involved in being with the parents after this event but was also very active in supporting all the midwifery and medical staff who had been involved in the woman's care. The following day the SHO was particularly distressed, as she blamed herself for the death of the baby. The chaplain was able to spend much time with her, helping her address the guilt and grief she was feeling.

The above case demonstrates that a chaplain can be helpful in providing support and counsel to both parents and staff in dealing with tragic events on the labour ward. How much a chaplain can be of use will depend on the relationship between him and those who work in this area and the issues of accessibility and communication. Deaths may occur very rapidly during labour and the use of a chaplain will depend on the ease and speed at which he may be contacted. In a busy, large hospital this may be very difficult. In others, having specific chaplains dedicated to working within the maternity unit means that they are readily accessible and that strong links are made with the staff.

Reflection: Have you had the experience of needing to contact a chaplain following a tragic event on the labour ward? Was he easy to contact and available?

Involvement in the postnatal period

After the birth of the child a chaplain may provide spiritual care in a number of ways. In the illustrations used above, where contact has been made in the antenatal period or labour, a chaplain will continue support into the postnatal period. However, he may also be available to those he has not cared for before. This will be a more common situation in UK trusts at the present time, where the majority of antenatal care now takes place in local communities and where hospital admissions are limited as much as possible. Some hospital trusts have chaplains dedicated to maternity units where regular visits are made to all areas. This makes it easier for midwifery and chaplaincy staff to get to know each other's working practices and to communicate about particular women's needs.

Some chaplaincies have also developed a thanksgiving service for the life of the new child, which takes place on a weekly basis. These services are meant to be non-threatening events designed for anyone to attend, whether they have a religious belief or not. In areas where the hospital chapel is well away from the maternity unit such services take place within the unit, using available space in tutorial or day rooms. This is more beneficial in that women can drop into the area without needing to make a special effort if they are very tired or not used to attending a religious service, and it enables them to bring their new baby as well. The disadvantage remains that attendance is reliant on the midwives giving information about the service in such a way that indicates it is open to everyone. This may be overcome to a certain extent by providing written invitations on admission to give information about when the service takes place, accompanied by clearly visible posters. However, personal reminders by enthusiastic staff on duty at the time will often encourage women to attend. Also, because it is often a weekly event, some women will miss out on the service due to the short time that they remain in hospital after the birth of the baby. Some will also find it hard to attend if they are unwell or undertaking examinations or tests at the time of the service. Recently, a friend commented on attending such a service some years previously. Though she was unable to remember the content, she recalled the value of it, enhanced by a card that was given to all the attendees as a reminder. This she had chosen to retain as a keepsake for her child for the future. Though this may originally have been thought of as a very simple gesture, it should be regarded as a valuable trigger to recalling the spiritual aspects of childbirth in the long term.

> *Reflection: How would you feel about having the opportunity to attend a thanksgiving service in your area? Would it be beneficial to the women in your care to know what takes place at such an event?*

Hospital chaplains may also have involvement in the postnatal period caring for the sick woman or infant. Within this context he may be able to provide counsel and support to the woman's family and to the staff concerned with her care, as well as meeting the needs of the woman herself. In a study of patients having experienced pregnancy loss, 64 per cent had visited the hospital chaplain for counsel, 67 per cent had asked for a blessing or baptism of the baby and 86 per cent had held some kind of memorial or funeral service (Heiman *et al.*, 1997). In this study, the patient's religiosity was not a factor in whether a funeral or memorial service was held, but was in relation to baptism. From this it can be suggested that the chaplain is a valuable support in caring for grieving parents. He may be specifically involved where babies are needing to be apart from their mothers on the neonatal unit and is also viewed as a major support to the staff who are caring for such patients (Burke and Matsumoto, 1999).

Case history 13

For an excellent illustration of the chaplain's work in relation to the neonatal unit the book *Holding On?*, a novel by Hazel McHaffie (1994), is to be recommended. Through the story of Peter, a preterm baby on life support, she explores the feelings and experiences of all those involved in his care. It includes exploration of some of the ethical, moral and spiritual issues surrounding the decisions relating to Peter's care. A complete chapter is dedicated to the role of the chaplain and clearly demonstrates some of the issues that may be raised in the daily life of a chaplain in a busy acute hospital, as well as his place in the life of a neonatal unit.

As with all issues relating to the neonatal unit, it is vital that there is effective communication between staff caring for the infant and those involved with the care of the woman, if she is still in hospital. This includes appropriate communication about the spiritual care that the infant has received and how the chaplain is involved. For instance, it is important to inform ward staff when an infant has received baptism or if a chaplain has needed to spend some time counselling a woman within the neonatal area. By ensuring such information is exchanged, continuity can be maintained with the appropriate chaplain. However, it is also important to ensure that no confidential information is given without the woman's consent.

In some units chaplains are responsible for holding memorial services for parents and staff to have the opportunity to remember the loss of particular infants (Small *et al.*, 1991). These may be held within the locality of the unit or away from the area in another building. Some chaplaincies have available a memorial book within a hospital chapel for prayers or messages to be written. The parents would then have the opportunity to come back and view the contents at any time.

Reflection: How may communication between community, ward and neonatal areas be improved in respect of spiritual care?

The woman's partner

For many couples the experiences of pregnancy and childbirth become opportunities for personal growth and development, sometimes as individuals and sometimes as a couple. With the bond of love that is generally present between couples who are having children it could be suggested that there will be a spiritual bond between them as well. Some women will thus rely on their partner to be their main source of spiritual support and comfort during pregnancy and childbirth, whether they have a religious belief or not. The spiritual qualities that may be particularly apparent in the partner could be:

- Enabling the woman's search for meaning.
- Love and compassion.
- Effective use of touch.

- Empathetic and intuitive behaviours.
- The ability to be present for the woman.

In the society in which we live, the partner could be either male or female, but it is unknown how significant this could be in the spiritual sense. There is no evidence to suggest that a spiritual bond between two women with one of them experiencing childbirth is any greater or less than that of a male and female who are undergoing the same. The female responses may be greater because of an ability to have a greater understanding or could be less due to the conflict in emotions that may be felt. For either gender, some partners will be spiritually strong enough to empower the woman whereas others will have the effect of diminishing her self-esteem. If this support is not available it may then become a source of conflict within a relationship. Spiritual support will vary from being religious, political or emotional and will vary in strength, depth and power, probably at different times of the pregnancy experience. The support will also be dependent on the partner's experience, culture and upbringing, personal faith and beliefs and their expectation of their role. This obviously makes the recognition of this support by a caring midwife very complicated! It is, however, realistic to expect that most couples will have some new/differing experiences in relation to personal growth during a pregnancy and that the partner will not always be available to the woman to be the source of support she needs. In a situation where the midwife has been able to get to know the family, she may be able to evaluate where there is conflict and provide spiritual support or guidance to both partners to enable such a conflict to be resolved. She may also be in a position to recognise the strengths present within the relationship and be able to further encourage a spiritual bond. However, in practical terms, this may be very difficult as it is rare for a midwife to be able to get to know both partners so intimately.

> *Reflection: Do you think it is realistic to expect a woman's partner to be her sole source of spiritual support during pregnancy?*

Antenatal issues

A knowledge of different cultures and beliefs is vital to understanding how a partner can influence a woman spiritually during her pregnancy. Schott and Henley's (1996) book provides a good source of information on cultures and religious belief in relation to childbirth. For many of the Jewish women in Sered's (1991) study, their husbands were regarded as being important for providing spiritual support in childbirth. They were expected to perform appropriate rituals that were thought to be more effective than the woman's own. Many of these women learned ritual from their husbands, and many expected the husband to consult the rabbi on the woman's behalf and then relate to her what the rabbi said to do. Within this context the need to perform religious rites follows on as a result of belief and birth within a particular culture. A midwife will need to be aware of religious rites that are used within the antenatal period and be encouraging and supportive to the partner to enable the couple to feel comfortable about continuing the practice. This may be easier within a woman's home, although it is important to create an hospital environment where people feel secure to maintain their religious integrity. The issue of privacy is important here and can lead to difficult situations in a busy hospital. The provision of a private area may be facilitated through the support of the hospital chaplain, and partners thus enabled to continue their religious practices. It is to be recognised that some cultures and religions view childbirth as 'women's work' and that it is normal practice for the male partner to choose to be excluded from involvement until after the event. In these situations the partner may be replaced by a close female relative acting as the woman's support.

As has already been discussed, not all women have religious faith, and there will be situations too where a partner's belief may be in conflict with the woman's. For instance, in the antenatal period upbringing and culture may have an influence on decision making regarding antenatal investigations or termination of the pregnancy for fetal abnormality. Differences in such beliefs may result in conflict over these decisions between partners. For the midwife involved there is a need for sensitivity and support, as well as enabling the woman to reach the right decision in these issues for her.

Reflection: Have you been aware in your practice of situations where there has been conflict between partners over moral or ethical decisions regarding the unborn child? How was this resolved?

For many women their partner may be a strength, enabling them to find meaning for themselves within the whole time of pregnancy. As they explore the issues that arise together, the partner may listen and help a woman to understand the emotions and conflicts that she has. Conversely, a partner may also create an atmosphere where the experience and/or her 'self' are devalued or undermined. It is realistic to expect that not all couples have strong, loving relationships, where a partner can meet a woman's innermost needs during pregnancy. It is also possible that a woman will want to search for meaning for herself outside of the relationship, which may result in conflict as she is unable to express herself deeply to her partner. For the midwife it may be difficult to become involved within these situations. In the first scenario she will be an observer outside of a strong relationship, while in the second she will be aware of tension developing. However, if she has been able to get to know the couple prior to the conflict developing, she may be able to intervene by aiding in issues of communication and encouraging the development of a greater spiritual bond. It is unrealistic to expect a midwife to be a counsellor in these situations, but it is possible to be supportive and a listener should either party wish to discuss such issues with her.

Labour involvement

Giving birth is an intimate event for women, despite the sad fact that so many do so within a highly technological hospital setting. Within this environment partners are still able to supply spiritual support through their intense presence – some through intuitive and empathetic means. Through their language they can support a woman through the experience and enable her to find spiritual meaning. The appropriate use of massage or a loving touch may also add a spiritual dimension to the birth. However, there is no doubt that many partners, and women, feel intimidated or threatened by a hospital setting and these support mechanisms may be enabled more appropriately within the couple's own home. Reading the birth stories of the couples in Ina May Gaskin's *Spiritual Midwifery* (1977) places in context the positive aspects of the presence of the partner at the birth. But it also indicates situations where the partner's presence is a hindrance to progress and where midwives have had the courage to ask the person to leave for a while. For many midwives this may be a very difficult thing to do, as they often do not meet the partner until the labour itself and, therefore, do not know what the person is like outside of the stressful situation in which they are placed.

Reflection: Have you been in situations where you wished you were able to ask the partner to leave the room for a while?

When the woman is in labour, partners may be involved in performing religious rites, often for the protection of the mother and baby. For instance, O'Shea's (1998) study revealed that prayer was regarded as important by couples for a safe delivery and for a perfect baby. She suggests that meaning may be brought into the act of giving birth by the reassurance of a religious belief. For one woman in the study, the importance of the partner being able to pray for the child immediately after the birth was significant to them. It is to be recognised that labour is a highly charged, emotional time for both partners, and some partners may find solace for themselves in continuing religious rituals, rather than providing support to the woman in labour. The midwife involved in this situation will need to be sensitive and be aware of the woman's responses to the partner. This again may be very difficult in the present hospital set-up of a midwife not knowing a couple before the event, and is more easily facilitated where a relationship has been developed in the antenatal period. A partner may also feel more able to act in an appropriate manner within their own home environment, and may feel more able to participate in ritual as required. The midwife may help to facilitate this by giving the couple privacy in labour at appropriate times and recognising when there is a need to leave them alone. A partner may also serve as a go-between in labour, providing information on progress to others who are aiming to give spiritual support through prayer. Keeping contact in this way will also enable the partner to be supported, especially if the labour is proving to be difficult.

Those who do not have a religious belief may find their spiritual support during labour in other ways such as through creative arts. For instance listening to or performing particular forms of music or reading poetry may prove relaxing. Others may need to perform other types of ritual. For some partners the need for the labour and birth to be normal may be regarded as a spiritual goal. Where the event then falls outside this desire, there may develop a conflict between the woman and her partner which in turn could lead to an experience of spiritual distress. The challenge for any midwife in these situations is to recognise what is important to each couple and establish effective and sensitive communication to ensure all needs are met.

Postnatal issues

Immediately following the birth there can be a surge of emotions and often gratitude for the safe arrival of the infant. This may frequently be accompanied by awe at the wonder of the creation of new life. During this time the partner may be involved in religious rites for the welcoming and safe arrival of the child, though these may take place later within the family's religious community. For the partner there may be a time of feeling something of an anticlimax as the woman and the baby often receive all the attention. This may be particularly marked when a partner has to leave to go home after a hospital birth. In some religious cultures, however, the male partner will receive all the adulation for the birth of the child, especially if it is a male child to carry on the family name (Schott and Henley, 1996).

Apart from religious rites that take place, partners may be involved in providing emotional and spiritual support postnatally through love and care, through effective touch to the new mother and baby, and through enabling the mother to find meaning in the experience. This may be more of a challenge if there are extra family members staying within the household. It is to be recognised that the addition of a child is a life-changing event for a partner as well as for a woman giving birth. It is during this time that it may be more difficult for the partner to be able to provide spiritual support to a woman, as they themselves are having to adjust emotionally and spiritually to a new life within the family. A change in their relationship, with the woman absorbed in caring for the needs of the baby, may mean that she is no longer so reliant on the partner to meet her spiritual needs. Emotionally the partner may feel excluded and may need to seek spiritual reassurance from elsewhere. A partner may experience a spiritual crisis after the birth, and this may be especially marked if the event has been traumatic or has lead to the loss of the infant or the woman. A midwife working with the couple may be able to recognise if this occurs and recommend the involvement of spiritual or religious advisors to give counsel as required.

Reflection: Have you been aware of partners who have appeared to experience trauma after the birth of their child? What mechanisms were/are in place to help them?

Friends and family

Magana and Clark's study (1995) suggested that being part of a community of believers may have a positive effect on the outcome of pregnancies through the social support and care given by those with the same beliefs and experiences. In their study, older women provided support through teaching on the best behaviour for the health and well-being of the unborn child. Though this was a study specifically based on a Mexican-American community, it is possible that there could be a positive effect for the pregnant woman living in any close-knit community where there was such influence from older women. However, this is dependent on the personal stance of the older women concerned and their own behaviour patterns. It should be pointed out that Magana and Clark's study was based in an area where religion had a particularly high focus, with accompanying positive behaviour patterns. Knowledge of what information is being provided by local religious groups is important. Midwives working in these communities can provide support through involvement in advising and educating on current advances in knowledge and care and encouraging positive health behaviours.

As indicated in previous chapters, some women are influenced to return to their family religious beliefs during pregnancy, possibly as a desire to belong. Certainly, the influence of the woman's mother in this is very strong. In some cultures this will involve the mother, along with other female relatives, taking over care of the woman completely following the birth, to the exclusion of the partner (Schott and Henley, 1996).

For some women spiritual growth and development will be through contacts and friendships, often started during pregnancy. Attendance at particular pregnancy preparation classes will lead to a spiritual need being met and special bonds being made. The influence may extend to the time of labour with the desire to have these friends as supporters. Knowledge of the woman's lifestyle and involvement is important for the midwife concerned in giving care, so that she may recognise the meaning and value the woman places on these friendships. Some midwives may find the intensity of these relationships a threat, especially if the friends serve to influence the choices the woman makes. Once again it is important to be sensitive to the woman's needs and wants and for there to be effective communication between all concerned.

> *Reflection: Have there been situations you have found difficult, where a woman's family or friends have attempted to influence her decisions and choices about her pregnancy or labour? Did the interference meet the woman's needs or was it detrimental? How did you respond? Would you respond differently now?*

Conclusion

It is clear from this chapter that a midwife will not be the only person to have an influence on the spiritual aspects of a woman's life during her pregnancy and birth. The influence of others, from formal religious leaders to partners, family and friends, will be very great and personal to her. There is a need to develop appropriate mechanisms to ensure that all are providing the correct spiritual support to the woman concerned, but it will take time and effort to establish how these mechanisms may be put in place. Individual midwives, with particular interest, may be influential in local communities in initiating communication with religious groups or local antenatal support networks. Others may be prepared to respond to individual's religious and spiritual needs within relationships. However, it is likely to be a long time before major inroads can be made that include all health carers concerned. The main need is to establish lines of effective communication between all involved and begin dialogue about pregnancy and birth, to understand what the spiritual needs may be. Working with partners, friends and family would be greatly assisted by getting to know the woman and her family set-up in the antenatal period and providing continuity for the labour and postnatally. Within these situations, as lead professional carer, a midwife would be well placed to ensure that the best possible spiritual care is given to the woman and her infant.

12 *Where do we go from here?*

It has been a challenge to write this book. It has been a journey of questioning and searching over a period of about 10 years, from my original thoughts as I watched others practise to now, where I watch others learn and develop to be midwives. During that time I have also changed and developed as a woman and experienced the joys and pains of motherhood four times. The contents of the book have also evolved with the development of my ideas and experiences and the welcome contribution of others. Even now there are further ways the book could be moved on. But there has to be an end. At the present time it seems wrong to call this chapter 'the conclusion'. Perhaps a better title would be 'the end of the beginning'. It is clear that this book has a number of weaknesses and limitations and there are too many constraints and difficulties in the subject matter to form an adequate conclusion. It is hoped, however, that the aims of provoking discussion and providing ideas for research will have been achieved.

Limitations

As it has been stated that there are limitations in this book, it is appropriate to reveal them to you. You may think there are some that may have been have missed! The lack of research and literature related to the spiritual care and spirituality of the pregnant woman has obviously made preparing this book a difficult process, and may even call into question its validity in our evidence-based culture! Also, the need to base the information on literature from mainly American sources may be regarded as a limitation. It is not known if there is a different perception of spirituality in different areas of the western world, or whether there is a perception of spirituality that is peculiar to the British population. Is it also right to label things as 'American' or 'British' anyway and assume that everyone within those countries are the same? My personal view would be to avoid such perceptions of culture and move towards individualizing care in all cases. This then makes research difficult! The need to base ideas mostly upon nursing research may also be regarded as a constraint, as the data may have been based on information from both male and female sources. The recognition of any differences in feminine and masculine approaches to spirituality would have to be important in addressing issues surrounding birth and midwifery care because of the naturally female slant to the experience. Those who are male midwives may find such a suggestion difficult but would perhaps recognize why this approach may be necessary.

The need to isolate the elements of spiritual issues in separate chapters is also a matter of concern. In truth, can we isolate all these things from each other, as there is so much overlap? Is it right to have isolated spirituality from the other aspects of a person – the body and mind? In true holistic care we would recognize the way in which all these aspects interact in a person and affect each other. If I am unwell in the physical sense it will have an effect on my psyche and my spiritual self. If I am unwell emotionally it will have an effect on me spiritually and I may exhibit physical symptoms. If I am unwell spiritually it will effect me physically and emotionally. Therefore, it would have been preferable not to split these elements of spirituality. But by not doing so, it would have been harder to illustrate that what midwives do already could be regarded as spiritual!

The way forward

There is a lot to do before we can say that we are meeting women's spiritual needs, according to the expectation of the rules of practice. There will be a need to shift our view on research and academia in order to effectively study spirituality. There will also need to be a shift in education in order to develop programmes that teach the subject effectively. Mostly there will need to be a move in the way midwives practise. This may be the biggest hurdle of all, as clinicians are battling against a poorly resourced system where they are already unable to meet women's needs. The expectation to be even more 'all-singing and all-dancing' midwives and to be spiritual as well may be too much for some!

However, with an end there also has to be a beginning. The aim of adding questions of reflection within the text was to aid this beginning. There were no right or wrong answers. By reading and reflecting on this book, hopefully it will have provoked discussion with others, and will lead to a snowball effect of ideas. It is hoped that researchers will be willing to take up the challenge of finding ways to study the process and for educators to discuss them with colleagues and students. Above all, it is hoped that practitioners of the art of midwifery will try changing their practice in little ways, and then reflect on these changes, assess if they help, and encourage others to do the same. By changing in small ways we can then have the confidence to change the big things that are hurdles to giving the best care.

Summary

The need for awareness and investigation of spirituality is important if midwives are going to provide holistic care. This book has highlighted elements of spiritual care that are already being carried out by midwives, and elements of spirituality that are experienced by pregnant and birthing women. Awareness of these issues should lead to establishing forms of care that will enhance the spiritual experience of the woman as well as encouraging midwives to give spiritual care. Through the information presented in this book it is suggested that the presence of a continuous relationship between a woman and a particular midwife is valuable and necessary for the effective provision of spiritual care. This relationship not only aids the midwife in giving effective spiritual care, but is also necessary to enable the woman to progress in her spiritual journey. Therefore, despite the limitations already explored, it is proposed that midwives should be aiming to continue to develop systems of practice that can encourage this special relationship to grow.

The future

The information in this book highlights the need for formal research into spiritual aspects related to the pregnant and birthing woman, and the spiritual care provided by midwives. The following areas are suggestions for studies in relation to spiritual care:

- Initially it may be appropriate to instigate a study to establish what are the elements of spiritual care given by midwives.
- The recognition that the establishment of an intense relationship between a woman and her midwife is a paramount feature of spiritual care would lead to the idea of a study to compare the spiritual aspects of care provided by midwives providing continuity and those who do not.
- Does religious belief in the midwife correlate with the provision of effective spiritual care? Does religious bias make a difference if the woman is not of the same belief?
- What are the characteristics of a spiritual midwife, perhaps based on Waugh's (1992) study relating to nurses' perceptions of spiritual care?
- Does the provision of spiritual care facilitate a 'normal' birth? In what way does it enhance the birth experience of the woman?
- How may midwives be encouraged to provide spiritual care through education? Is spiritual care a subject that can be taught, or is it something within a particular midwife?

In relation to the woman's spirituality, the following may be studied:

- What is a woman's awareness and response to spiritual aspects antenatally, during labour and postnatally?
- What are a woman's spiritual needs and how may a midwife meet them?
- What significance does religious belief have to the woman during pregnancy and birth, and what effect does spirituality have upon the 'normality' and ease of birth?
- A comparison of women with different beliefs before pregnancy, and how these are affected by, or have an effect on, the birth experience.
- Is there a difference between the spiritual needs and awareness of women with belief and those without?
- What factors are important in recognizing those women who may be at risk of spiritual distress and how may they be cared for effectively?
- How does the growth in spiritual awareness affect the relationship with the child and the adaptation of the woman to motherhood?

References

Achterberg, J. (1990) *Woman as Healer*. Rider.

Allen, C. (1991) The inner light. *Nursing Standard*, **5**(20), 52–53.

Allott, H. (1996) Picking up the pieces: the post-delivery stress clinic. *British Journal of Midwifery*, **4**(10), 534–536.

Amenta, M.O. (1997) Spiritual care: the heart of palliative nursing. *International Journal of Palliative Nursing*, **3**(1), 4.

Annandale, E. and Clark, J. (1996) What is gender? Feminist theory and the sociology of human reproduction. *Sociology of Health and Illness*, **18**(1), 17–44.

Atkins, A. (1998) *Split Image: Discovering God's True Intention for Male and Female*. Hodder and Stoughton.

Baginsky, Y. (1986) I am a woman who carries a child. In *Birth Matters: Issues and Alternatives in Childbirth* (R. Claxton, ed.). Unwin Paperbacks.

Balin, J. (1988) The sacred dimensions of pregnancy and birth. *Qualitative Sociology*, **11**(4), 275–301.

Ball, J. (1994) *Reactions to Motherhood – The Role of Postnatal Care*, 2nd Edn. Books for Midwives Press.

Bates, C. (1997) Care in normal labour; a feminist perspective. In *Midwifery Practice: Core Topics 2* (J. Alexander, V. Levy and C. Roth, eds). Macmillan Press.

Beech, B. (1986) Know your rights: a parents' guide to birth. In *Birth Matters: Issues and Alternatives in Childbirth* (R. Claxton, ed.). Unwin Paperbacks.

Belbin, A. (1996) Power and choice in birthgiving: a case study. *British Journal of Midwifery*, **4**(5), 264–267.

Belenky, M., Clinchy, B., Goldberger, M. *et al.* (1986) *Women's Ways of Knowing: The Development of Self, Voice and Mind*. Basic Books Inc.

Berg, M., Lundgren, I., Hermansson, E. *et al.* (1996) Women's experience of the encounter with the midwife during childbirth. *Midwifery*, **12**, 11–15.

Berg, M. and Dahlberg, K. (1998) A phenomenological study of women's experiences of complicated childbirth. *Midwifery*, **14**, 23–29.

Bergum, V. (1989) *Woman to Mother: A Transformation*. Bergin andGarvey Publishers Inc.

Berryman, J.C. and Windridge, K.C. (1995) *Motherhood after 35: A report on the Leicester Motherhood project*. Leicester University and Nestlé.

Bloom, M. (1981) The romance and power of breastfeeding. *Birth and The Family Journal*, **8**(4), 259–269.

Bluff, R. and Holloway, I. (1994) 'They know best': Women's perceptions of midwifery care during labour and childbirth. *Midwifery*, **10**, 157–164.

Bottorff, J.L. (1991) The lived experience of being comforted by a nurse. *Phenomenology and Pedagogy*, **9**, 237–252.

Boutell, K.A. and Bozett, F.W. (1990) Nurses' assessment of patients' spirituality: Continuing education implications. *The Journal of Continuing Education in Nursing*, **21**(4), 172–176.

Bradshaw, A. (1997) Teaching spiritual care to nurses: An alternative approach. *International Journal of Palliative Nursing*, **3**(1), 51–57.

Brady-Fryer, B. (1994) Becoming the mother of a preterm baby. In *Uncertain Motherhood: Negotiating The Risks of The Childbearing Years* (P.A. Field and P.B. Marck, eds). Sage Publications.

Brown, C.K. (1998) The integration of healing and spirituality into health care. *Journal of Interprofessional Care*, **12**(4), 373–381.

Brown, Y. (1993) Perinatal loss: A framework for practice. *Health Care for Women International*, **14**, 469–479.

Brown-Saltzman, K. (1997) Replenishing the spirit by meditative prayer and guided imagery. *Seminars in Oncology Nursing*, **13**(4), 255–259.

Burke, S.S. and Matsumoto, A.R. (1999) Pastoral care for perinatal and neonatal health care providers. *JOGNN*, **28**, 137–141.

Burkhardt, M.A. (1994) Becoming and connecting: Elements of spirituality for women. *Holistic Nursing Practice*, **8**(4), 12–21.

Burkhardt, M.A. (1998) Reintegrating spirituality into healthcare. *Alternative Therapies*, **4**(2), 128–127.

Burnard, P. (1988) Searching for meaning. *Nursing Times*, **84**(37), 34/36.

Callister, L.C. (1995) Cultural meanings of childbirth. *Journal of Obstetric, Gynaecologic and Neonatal Nursing*, **24**(4), 327–331.

Callister, L.C., Vehvilainen-Julkunen, K. and Lauri, S. (1996) Cultural perceptions of childbirth: A cross-cultural comparison of childbearing women. *Journal of Holistic Nursing*, **14**(1), 66–78.

Carson, V.B. (1989a) Spirituality and the nursing process. In *Spiritual Dimensions of Nursing Practice* (V.B. Carson, ed.). W.B. Saunders Co.

Carson, V.B. (1989b) Spiritual development across the life span. In *Spiritual Dimensions of Nursing Practice* (V.B. Carson, ed.). W.B. Saunders Co.

Catterall, R.A., Cox, M., Greet, B. *et al.* (1998) The assessment and audit of spiritual care. *International Journal of Palliative Nursing*, **4**(4), 162–168.

Cawley, N. (1997) An exploration of the concept of spirituality. *International Journal of Palliative Nursing*, **3**(1), 31–36.

Chesney, M. (1996) Sharing reflections on critical incidents in midwifery practice. *British Journal of Midwifery*, **4**(1), 8–11.

Childbirth and Parenting Ministries (1999) URL: www.onfire.org.au/hilbig/cpm.htm.

Clark, C.C., Cross, J.R., Deane, D.M. *et al.* (1991) Spirituality: Integral to quality care. *Holistic Nursing Practice*, **5**(3), 67–76.

Clarke, R. (1996) All you need is love. *Modern Midwife*, **6**(7), 30.

Clarke, J.B. and Wheeler, S.J. (1992) A view of the phenomenon of caring in nursing practice. *Journal of Advanced Nursing*, **17**, 1283–1290.

Cohen, J.(1996) Integrating water into maternity care. *Midwifery Today*, **39**, 36.

Corrine, L., Bailey, V., Valentin, M. *et al.* (1992) The unheard voices of women: Spiritual interventions in maternal-child health. *American Journal of Maternal Child Nursing*, **17**(3), 141–145.

Cusveller, B.S. (1995) A view from somewhere: The presence and function of religious commitment in nursing practice. *Journal of Advanced Nursing*, **22**, 973–978.

Cusveller, B.S. (1998) Cut from the right wood: Spiritual and ethical pluralism in professional nursing practice. *Journal of Advanced Nursing*, **28**(2), 266–273.

Daaleman, T.P. and Nease, D.E. (1994) Patient attitudes regarding physician inquiry into spiritual and religious issues. *Journal of Family Practice*, **39**(6), 564–568.

Dally, A. (1982) *Inventing Motherhood: The Consequences of An Ideal.* Barrett Books Ltd.

Davies, C. (1997) When a baby dies. *Nursing Times*, **93**(8), 28–29.

Davies, D. (1994) Introduction: Raising the issues. In *Rites of Passage* (J. Holm and J. Bowker, eds) Pinter Publishers Ltd.

Davis, D. (1995) Ways of knowing in midwifery. *Australian College of Midwives Incorporated Journal*, **8**(3), 30–32.

Davis, L. (1996) Opportunity knocks. *The Cord*, (4), 5–7, New Arrivals.

Davis-Floyd, R. and Davis, E. (1997) Intuition as authoritative knowledge in midwifery and home birth. In *Childbirth and Authoritative Knowledge: Cross-cultural Perspectives* (R. Davis Floyd and C.F. Sargent, eds). Berkley Press.

Department of Health, Expert Maternity Group (1993) *Changing Childbirth, Part 1.* HMSO.

Diachuk, M.G. (1994) When a child has a birth defect. In *Uncertain Motherhood: Negotiating the Risks of the Childbearing Years* (P.A. Field and P.B. Marck, eds). Sage Publications.

Dickinson, C. (1975) The search for spiritual meaning. *American Journal of Nursing*, **75**(10), 1789–1793.

Dobbie, B.J. (1991) Women's mid-life experience: an evolving consciousness of self and children. *Journal of Advanced Nursing*, **16**, 825–831.

Dombeck, M.B. (1995) Dream telling: A means of spiritual awareness. *Holistic Nursing Practice*, **9**(2), 37–47.

Dombeck, M.T. (1998) The spiritual and pastoral dimensions of care in interprofessional contexts. *Journal of Interprofessional Care*, **12**(4), 361–371.

Downe, S. (1998) Motherless mothers and social support. *British Journal of Midwifery*, **6**(10), 682.

Edassery, D. and Kuttierath, S.K. (1998) Spirituality in the secular sense. *European Journal of Palliative Care*, **5**(5), 165–167.

Edmunds, J. (1995) The journey-dance of labor and birth. *Midwifery Today*, **33**, 54.

Eisenstein, H. (1984) *Contemporary Feminist Thought*. Unwin Paperbacks.

Estes, C.P. (1992) *Women Who Run With The Wolves*. Rider Books.

Evans, F. (1991) The Newcastle community midwifery care project. Part 2: The evaluation of the project. In *Midwives, Research and Childbirth, Vol. II* (S. Robinson and A.M. Thomson, eds) Chapman and Hall.

Fish, S. and Shelly, J.A. (1978) *Spiritual Care: The Nurse's Role*. Intervarsity Press.

Flagler, S. and Nicoll, L. (1990) A framework for the psychological aspects of pregnancy, NAACOGS. *Clinical Issues of Perinatal and Women's Health Nursing*, **1**(3), 297–302.

Flint, C. (1986) *Sensitive Midwifery*. Heinemann Midwifery.

Flint, C. and Poulengeris, P. (1987) *The 'Know Your Midwife' Report*, available from 49 Peckarmans Wood, London SE26 6RZ.

Fraser, J. (1997) *Child Protection – A Guide for Midwives*. Books for Midwives Press.

Gaskin, I.M. (1977) *Spiritual Midwifery*. The Book Publishing Co.

Gittens, D. (1985) *The Family in Question*. Macmillan Press.

Goddard, N.C. (1995) 'Spirituality as integrative energy': A philosophical analysis as requisite precursor to holistic nursing practice. *Journal of Advanced Nursing*, **22**, 808–815.

Goodenough, T. and Barratt, J. (1991) *Midwives' and mothers' perceptions of the transition to parenthood*. PhD Thesis, University of Bristol.

Guinness, M. (1993) *Tapestry of voices – meditations on women's lives*. Triangle.

Hall, J. (1990) A hard decision – the psychological effects of termination on a subsequent pregnancy. *Nursing Times*, **86**(47), 33–35.

Hall, C. and Lanig, H. (1993) Spiritual caring behaviors as reported by Christian nurses. *Western Journal of Nursing Research*, **15**(6), 730–741.

Halldorsdottir, S. and Karlsdottir, S.I. (1996) Empowerment or discouragement: Women's experience of caring and uncaring encounters during childbirth. *Health Care for Women International*, **17**, 361–379.

Hampton, M.R. (1995) Searching for their roots in birth. *Midwifery Today*, **33**, 14–15, 40.

Harris, R.E. (1994) The process of infertility. In *Uncertain Motherhood: Negotiating The Risks of The Childbearing Years* (P.A. Field and P.B. Marck, eds). Sage Publications.

Harrison, J. (1993) Spirituality and nursing practice. *Journal of Clinical Nursing*, **2**, 211–217.

Harrison, J. and Burnard, P. (1993) *Spirituality and Nursing Practice*. Avebury.

Hebblethwaite, M. (1984) *Motherhood and God*. Geoffrey Chapman Books.

Heiman, J., Yankowitz, J. and Wilkins, J. (1997) Grief support program: patients' use of services following the loss of a desired pregnancy and degree of implementation in academic centers. *American Journal of Perinatology*, **14**(10), 587–591.

Hernes, G. (1996) The politics of health of women and children. *Midwifery*, **12**, 109–112.

Hicks, C. (1993) Effects of psychological prejudices on communication and social interaction. *British Journal of Midwifery*, **1**(1), 10–16.

Highfield, M. and Cason, C. (1983) Spiritual needs of patients Are they recognised? *Cancer Nursing*, **6**, 187–192.

Hillyer, C. (1987) A personal experience of a home birth in California attended by two lay-midwives. *Association of Radical Midwives Magazine*, **33**, 16–17.

Holm, J. and Bowker, J. (1994a) *Women in Religion*. Pinter Publishing Ltd.

Holm, J. and Bowker, J. (1994b) *Rites of Passage*. Pinter Publishing Ltd.

Hunt, M.E. (1995) Psychological implications of women's spiritual health. *Women and Therapy*, **16**(2/3), 21–32.

Hunt, S. and Symonds, A. (1995) *The Social Meaning of Midwifery*. Macmillan Press.

Illsley, R. and Hall, M.H. (1976) *Psychosocial aspects of abortion*. WHO Bulletin 53, 83–106.

James, S. (1995) Gossip, stories and friendship: Confidentiality in midwifery practice. *Nursing Ethics*, **2**(4), 295–302.

Jenner, S. (1988) The influence of additional information advice and support on the success of breastfeeding in working class primiparas. *Child: Care, Health and Development*, **14**, 319–328.

Jones, A.W. (1990) A survey of general practioners' attitudes to the involvement of clergy in patient care. *British Journal of General Practice*, **40**, 280–283.

Kahn, R.P. (1995) *Bearing Meaning: The Language of Birth*. University of Illinois Press.

Kaye, J. and Robinson, K.M. (1994) Spirituality among caregivers. *IMAGE Journal of Nursing Scholarship*, **26**(3), 218–221.

Keighley, T. (1997) Organisational structures and personal spiritual belief. *International Journal of Palliative Nursing*, **3**(1), 51–57.

Kennell, J., Klaus, M. McGrath, S. *et al.* (1991) Continuous emotional support during labor in a US hospital. *Journal of the American Medical Association*, **265**(17), 2197–2201.

Khalaf, I. and Callister, L.C. (1997) Cultural meanings of childbirth; Muslim women living in Jordan. *Journal of Holistic Nursing*, **15**(4), 373–388.

King, U. (1993) *Women and Spirituality*, 2nd Edn. Macmillan Press.

Kirkham, M.J. (1989) Midwives and information-giving during labour. In *Midwives, Research and Childbirth, Vol. 1* (S. Robinson and A.M. Thomson, eds). Chapman and Hall.

Kirkham, M.J. (1997) Stories and childbirth. In *Reflections on Midwifery* (M.J. Kirkham and E.R. Perkins, eds). Bailliere Tindall.

Kitzinger, S.(1989) Childbirth and society. In *Effective Care in Pregnancy and Childbirth* (I. Chalmers, M. Enkin and J.N.C. Keirse, eds). Oxford University Press.

Kitzinger, S. (1997) Authoritative touch in childbirth – a cross-cultural approach. In *Childbirth and Authoritative Knowledge: Cross-cultural Perspectives* (R.E. Davis-Floyd and C.F. Sargent, eds). Berkley Press.

Klaus, M.H., Kennell, J.H., Robertson, S.S. *et al.* (1986) Effects of social support during parturition on maternal and infant morbidity. *British Medical Journal*, **293**(6547), 585–587.

Labun, E. (1988) Spiritual care: An element in nursing care planning. *Journal of Advanced Nursing*, **13**, 314–320.

LaChance, C.W. (1991) *The Way Of The Mother*. Element Books Ltd.

Lane, J. (1987) The care of the human spirit. *Journal of Professional Nursing*, **3**, 332–337.

Laryea, M. (1989) Midwives' and mothers' perceptions of motherhood. In *Midwives, Research and Childbirth, Vol. 1* (S. Robinson and A.M. Thomson, eds). Chapman and Hall.

Lavender, T. and Walkinshaw, S.A. (1998) Can midwives reduce postpartum psychological morbidity? A randomized trial. *Birth*, **25**(4), 215–219.

Lovell, A. (1996) Power and choice in birthgiving: some thoughts. *British Journal of Midwifery*, **4**(5), 268–272.

Lundgren, I. and Dahlberg, K. (1998) Women's experience of pain during childbirth. *Midwifery*, **14**, 105–110.

Macnutt, F. and Macnutt, J. (1988) *Praying For Your Unborn Child*. Hodder and Stoughton.

Magana, A. and Clark, N.M. (1995) Examining a paradox: Does religiosity contribute to positive birth outcomes in Mexican American populations? *Health Education Quarterly*, **22**(1), 96–109.

Marck, P.B. (1994) Unexpected pregnancy: the uncharted land of women's experience. In *Uncertain Motherhood: Negotiating The Risks of The Childbearing Years* (P.A. Field and P.B. Marck, eds). Sage Publications.

Marck, P.B., Field, P.A. and Bergum, V. (1994) A search for understanding. In *Uncertain Motherhood: Negotiating The Risks of The Childbearing Years* (P.A. Field and P.B. Marck, eds). Sage Publications.

Mason, J. (1990) The meaning of birth stories. *The Birth Gazette*, **6**(3), 14–19.

McCool, W.F. and McCool, S.J. (1989) Feminism and nurse-midwifery-historical overview and current issues. *Journal of Nurse-midwifery*, **34**(6), 323–334.

McHaffie, H. (1994) *Holding On?* Books for Midwives Press.

McGeary, K. (1994) The influence of guarding on the developing mother-unborn child relationship. In *Uncertain Motherhood: Negotiating The Risks of The Childbearing Years* (P.A. Field and P.B. Marck, eds). Sage Publications.

McGilloway, O. (1985) Religious beliefs, practices, and philosophies. In *Nursing and Spiritual Care* (O. McGilloway and F. Myco, eds). Harper and Row Publishers Ltd.

Mckay, S. (1991) Shared power: The essence of humanized childbirth. *Pre- and Peri-natal Psychology*, **5**(4), 283–295.

McSherry, W. (1996) Raising the spirits. *Nursing Times*, **92**(3), 48–49.

McSherry, W. and Draper, P. (1997) The spiritual dimension: Why the absence within nursing curricula? *Nursing Education Today*, **17**, 413–417.

Menage, J. (1996) Post-traumatic stress disorder following obstetric/gynaecological procedures. *British Journal of Midwifery*, **4**(10), 532–533.

Midwives' Alliance of North America (MANA) (1992) MANA statement of core values and ethics, *MANA News*, **10**(4), 10–12.

Moberg, D.O. (1979) The development of social indicators of spiritual well-being for quality of life research. In *Spiritual Well-being – Sociological Perspectives* (D.O. Moberg, ed.). University Press of America.

Morgan, M. (1996) Prenatal care of African American women in selected USA urban and rural cultural contexts. *Journal of Transcultural Nursing*, **7**(2), 3–9.

Morris, D. (1991) *Babywatching*. Jonathan Cape Press.

Murphy, F. and Hunt, S. (1997) Early pregnancy loss: Men have feelings too. *British Journal of Midwifery*, 5(2), 87–90.

Murray, R.R. and Zentner, J.P. (1989) *Nursing Concepts For Health Promotion*. Prentice Hall.

Myco, F. (1985) The non-believer in the health care situation. In *Nursing and Spiritual Care* (O. McGilloway and F. Myco, eds). Harper and Row.

NANDA (1994) *Nursing Diagnosis*. NANDA.

Najman, J.M., Williams, G.M., Keeping, J.D. *et al.* (1988) Religious values, practices and pregnancy outcomes: A comparison of the impact of sect and mainstream Christian affiliation. *Social Science and Medicine*, **26**(4), 401–407.

Narayanasamy, A. (1993) Nurses' awareness and educational preparation in meeting their patients' spiritual needs. *Nurse Education Today*, **13**, 196–201.

Nichols, F.H. (1996) The meaning of the childbirth experience: A review of the literature. *The Journal of Perinatal Education*, **5**(4), 71–77.

Oakley, A. (1992) *Social Support and Motherhood*. Blackwell Press.

Odent, M. (1984) *Birth Reborn*. Souvenir Press.

Odent, M. (1994) The love hormones. *Primal Health Research*, **2**(3), 3–7.

Oldnall, A. (1996) A critical analysis of nursing: Meeting the spiritual needs of patients. *Journal of Advanced Nursing*, **23**, 138–144.

Olsen, D.P. (1991) Empathy as an ethical and philosophical basis for nursing. *Advances in Nursing Science*, **14**(1), 62–75.

O'Shea, M. (1998) *An exploratory study of women's experience of childbirth specifically identifying the spiritual dimension*. Dissertation for BSc Midwifery Studies, The Nightingale Institute, King's College, London.

Osterman, P. and Schwartz-Barcott, D. (1996) Presence: four ways of being there. *Nursing Forum*, 31(2), 23–30.

Page, L. (1993) Redefining the midwife's role: changes needed in practice. *British Journal of Midwifery*, **1**(1), 21–24.

Page, L. (1996) Positive care in childbirth. *British Journal of Midwifery*, **4**(10), 530–532.

Parvati Baker, J. (1993) Wombside earthside. *Compleat Mother*, Fall, 18–19.

Paykel, E.S., Emms, E.M., Fletcher, J. *et al.* (1980) Life events and social support in puerperal depression. *British Journal of Psychiatry*, **136**, 339–346.

Penwell, V. (1996) Power for healing. *The Cord*, **4**, 18–19 New Arrivals.

Praill, D. (1995) Approaches to spiritual care. *Nursing Times*, **91**(34), 55–57.

Price, J. (1988) *Motherhood – What It Does To Your Mind*. Pandora Press.

Price, J.L., Stevens, H.O. and LaBarre, M.C. (1995) Spiritual caregiving in nursing practice. *Journal of Psychosocial Nursing*, **33**(12), 5–9.

Priya, J.V. (1992) *Birth Traditions and Modern Pregnancy Care*. Element Books Ltd.

Raphael-Leff, J. (1991) *Psychological Processes of Childbearing*. Chapman and Hall.

Raphael-Leff, J. (1993) *Pregnancy –The Inside Story*. Sheldon Press.

Rawlings, L. (1995) Re-imagining birth. *Birth Gazette*, **11**(4), 14–17.

Reading, A.E. and Cox, D.N. (1982) The effect of ultrasound examination on maternal anxiety levels. *Journal of Behavioural Medicine*, **5**, 237–247.

Reed, P.G. (1986) Religiousness among terminally ill and healthy adults. *Research in Nursing and Health*, **9**, 35–41.

Rew, L. (1989) Intuition: Nursing knowledge and the spiritual dimension of persons. *Holistic Nursing Practice*, **3**(3), 56–68.

Rhodes, J. (1997) The wild goose: female spirituality and counselling. *Contact: The Interdisciplinary Journal of Pastoral Studies*, **124**, 24–27.

Rich, A. (1992) *Of Woman Born – Motherhood as Experience and Institution*, 2nd Edn. Virago Press Ltd.

Richardson, D. (1993) *Women, Motherhood and Childrearing*. Macmillan Press.

Ross, L.A. (1994) Spiritual aspects of nursing. *Journal of Advanced Nursing*, **19**, 439–447.

Ross, L.A. (1996) Teaching spiritual care to nurses. *Nurse Education Today*, **16**, 38–43.

Ross, L. (1997) The nurse's role in assessing and responding to patients' spiritual needs. *International Journal of Palliative Nursing*, **3**(1), 37–42.

Rothman, B.K. (1994) *The Tentative Pregnancy – Amnoicentesis and The Sexual Politics of Motherhood*. Pandora Press.

Rubin, R. (1984) *Maternal Identity and Maternal Experience*. Springer Publishing Co.

Salter, J. (1987) *The Incarnating Child*. Hawthorn Press.

Sandall, J. (1997) Midwives' burnout and continuity of care. *British Journal of Midwifery*, **5**(2), 106–111.

Savett, L.A. (1997) Spirituality and practice: Stories, barriers and opportunities. *Creative Nursing*, **3**(4), 7–11, 16.

Sayers, J. (1989) Childbirth: Patriarchal and maternal influences. *Journal of Reproductive and Infant Psychology*, **7**, 15–24.

Schott, J. and Henley, A. (1996) *Culture, Religion and Childbearing in a Multiracial Society*. Butterworth-Heinemann.

Schwartz, L. (1991) *Bonding Before Birth*. Sigo Press.

Sered, S.S. (1991) Childbirth as a religious experience? Voices from an Israeli hospital. *Journal of Feminist Studies in Religion*, 7(2), 7–18.

Sered, S.S. (1994) *Priestess, Mother, Sacred Sister: Religions Dominated by Women*. Oxford University Press.

Sherr, L. (1995) *The Psychology of Pregnancy and Childbirth*. Blackwell Science Ltd.

Siddiqui, J. (1999) The therapeutic relationship in midwifery. *British Journal of Midwifery*, **7**(2), 111–114.

Silverton, L. (1993) *The Art and Science of Midwifery*. Prentice Hall International (UK) Ltd.

Simkin, P. (1991) Just another day in a woman's life? Women's long-term perceptions of their first birth experience. Part 1. *Birth*, **18**(4), 203–210.

Sims, A. (1994) 'Psyche' – spirit as well as mind? *British Journal of Psychiatry*, 165, 441–446.

Simsen, B. (1988) Nursing the spirit. *Nursing Times*, **84**(37), 31–33.

Singh Kalsi, S. (1994) Sikhism. In *Rites of Passage* (J. Holm and J. Bowker, eds). Pinter Publishers Ltd.

Small, M., Engler, A.J. and Rushton, C. H. (1991) Saying goodbye in the intensive care unit: Helping caregivers grieve. *Pediatric Nursing*, **17**(1), 103–105.

Smith, J.A. and Mitchell, S. (1996) Debriefing after childbirth: A tool for effective risk management. *British Journal of Midwifery*, **4**(11), 581–586.

Smucker, C. (1996) A phenomenological description of the experience of spiritual distress. *Nursing Diagnosis*, **7**(2), 81–91.

Snijders, R.J.M., Noble, P., Sebire, N. *et al.* (1998) UK multicentre project on assessment of risk of trisomy 21 by maternal age and fetal nuchal translucency thickness at 10–14 weeks gestation. *Lancet*, **352**(9125), 343–346.

Sodestrom, K.E. and Martinson, I.M. (1987) Patients' spiritual coping strategies: A study of nurse and patient perspectives. *Oncology Nurses Forum*, **14**(2), 41–46.

Sokoloski, E.H. (1995) Canadian First Nations women's beliefs about pregnancy and prenatal care. *Canadian Journal of Nursing Research*, **27**(1), 89–100.

Soskice, J.M. (1992) Can a feminist call God 'Father'? In *Women's Voices: Essays in Contemporary Theology* (T. Elwes, ed.). Marshall Pickering.

Sosa, R., Kennel, J., Klaus, M. *et al.* (1980) The effect of a supportive companion on perinatal problems, length of labor, and mother–infant interaction. *The New England Journal of Medicine*, **303**(11), 597–600.

Sowell, R.L. and Misener, T.R. (1997) Decisions to have a baby by HIV-infected women. *Western Journal of Nursing Research*, **19**(1), 56–70.

Speck, P. (1988) *Being There*. SPCK.

Stanworth, R. (1997) Spirituality, language and depth of reality. *International Journal of Palliative Nursing*, **3**(1), 19–22.

Stockley, S. (1986) Psychic and spiritual aspects of pregnancy, birth and life. In *Birth Matters* (R. Claxton, ed.). Unwin Paperbacks.

Stoll, R.I. (1979) Guidelines for spiritual assessment. *American Journal of Nursing*, **79**, 1579–1587.

Stoll, R.I. (1989) The essence of spirituality. In *Spiritual Dimensions of Nursing Practice* (V.B. Carson, ed.). W.B. Saunders Co.

Stone, J. (1993) Whose pregnancy is it anyway? *Health Matters*, **16**, 12–13.

Storkey, E. (1985) *What's Right With Feminism*. SPCK.

Sugirtharajah, S. (1994) Hinduism. In *Women in Religion* (J. Holm and J. Bowker, eds). Pinter Publishers Ltd.

Sumner, C.H. (1998) Recognizing and responding to spiritual distress. *American Journal of Nursing*, **98**(1), 26–30.

Sykes, J.B. (ed.)(1977) *The Concise Oxford Dictionary*, 6th Edn. Book Club Associates.

Taylor, E.J. (1997) The story behind the story: the use of storytelling in spiritual caregiving. *Seminars in Oncology Nursing*, **13**(4), 252–254.

Thomson, A.M. (1981) Stillbirth. *Contact*, **72**(3), 2–9.

Tucakovic, M. (1994) Spiritual aesthetics in nursing. *The Australian Journal of Holistic Nursing*, **1**(1), 16–27.

UKCC (1993) Midwives Rules. UKCC for Nursing, Midwifery and Health Visiting.

Underdown, A. (1998) The transition to parenthood. *British Journal of Midwifery*, **6**(8), 508–511.

VandeCreek, L.(1997) Collaboration between nurses and chaplains for spiritual caregiving. *Seminars in Oncology Nursing*, **13**(4), 279–280.

Verny, T. and Kelly, J. (1982) *The Secret Life of The Unborn Child*. Sphere Books.

Wagner, V. (1995) Question of the quarter. *Midwifery Today*, **33**, 26.

Waugh, L.A. (1992) *Spiritual aspects of nursing: A descriptive study of nurses' perceptions*. PhD Thesis, Queen Margaret College, Edinburgh.

Wikman, M., Jacobsson, L., von Schoultz, B. (1992) Attitudes toward reproduction in a nonpatient population. *American Journal of Obstetrics and Gynaecology*, **166**, 121–126.

Wright, A. (1994) Judaism. In *Women in Religion* (J. Holm and J. Bowker, eds). Pinter Publishers Ltd.

Yao, X. (1994) Chinese religion. In *Rites of Passage* (J. Holm and J. Bowker, eds). Pinter Publishers Ltd.

Yearley, C. (1997) Motherhood as a rite of passage: An anthropological perspective. In *Midwifery Practice: Core Topics 2* (J. Alexander, V. Levy and C. Roth, eds). Macmillan Press.

Index